"When you arise in the morning, think what a precious privilege it is to live, to breathe, to think, to enjoy, to love." --MARCUS AURELIUS.

"Nature Cures" --HIPPOCRATES

TO ISAAC T. COOK

WHOSE CRITICISMS, ASSISTANCE AND ENCOURAGEMENT HAVE LIGHTENED THE LABOR AND ADDED TO THE PLEASURE OF PRODUCING THIS VOLUME.

CHAPTER CONTENTS

I PRELIMINARY CONSIDERATIONS Humanity, Health and Healers

II MENTAL ATTITUDE Correct and Incorrect--Results

III FOOD General Consideration

IV OVEREATING

V DAILY FOOD INTAKE

VI WHAT TO EAT

VII WHEN TO EAT

VIII HOW TO EAT

IX CLASSIFICATION OF FOODS

X FLESH FOODS Composition--Utility--Preparation--Combinations

XI NUTS Composition--Utility--Preparation--Combinations

XII LEGUMES Composition--Utility--Preparation--Combinations

XIII SUCCULENT VEGETABLES Composition--Utility--Preparation--Combinations--Salads

XIV CEREAL FOODS Composition--Utility--Preparation--Combinations

XV TUBERS Composition--Utility--Preparation--Combinations

XVI FRUITS Composition--Utility--Preparation--Combinations--Salads

XVII OILS AND FATS

XVIII MILK AND OTHER DAIRY PRODUCTS Composition--Utility--Preparation--

Combinations

XIX MENUS Food Combination in General

XX DRINK Water--Tea--Coffee--Alcohol--Enslaving Drugs

XXI CARE OF THE SKIN Baths--Friction--Clothing

XXII EXERCISE

XXIII BREATHING AND VENTILATION

XXIV SLEEP

XXV FASTING Our Most Important Remedy--Symptoms--When and How to Fast--Cases

XXVI ATTITUDE OF PARENT TOWARD CHILD

XXVII CHILDREN Prenatal Care--Infancy--Childhood--Mental Training

XXVIII DURATION OF LIFE Advanced Years--Living to Old Age in Health and Comfort

XXIX EVOLVING INTO HEALTH How it is Often Done--A Case

XXX RETROSPECT A Summing-up of the Subject

CHAPTER I.

PRELIMINARY CONSIDERATIONS.

Writings on hygiene and health have been accessible for centuries, but never before have books and magazines on these subjects been as numerous as they are today. Most of the information is so general, vague and indefinite that only a few have the time and patience to read the thousands of pages necessary to learn what to do to keep well. The truth is to be found in the archives of medicine, in writings covering a period of over thirty centuries, but it is rather difficult to find the grains of truth.

Health is the most valuable of all possessions, for with health one can attain anything else within reason. A few of the great people of the world have been sickly, but it takes men and women sound in body and mind to do the important work. Healthy men and women are a nation's most valuable asset.

It is natural to be healthy, but we have wandered so far astray that disease is the rule and good health the exception. Of course, most people are well enough to attend to their work, but nearly all are suffering from some ill, mental or physical, acute or chronic, which deprives them of a part of their power. The average individual is of less value to himself, to his family and to society than he could be. His bad habits, of which he is often not aware, have brought weakness and disease upon him. These conditions prevent him from doing his best mentally and physically.

This abnormal condition has a bad effect upon his descendants, who may not be born with any special defects, but they have less resistance at birth than is their due, and consequently fall prey to disease very easily. This state of impaired resistance has been passed on from generation to generation, and we of today are passing it on as a heritage to our children.

About 280,000 babies under the age of one year die annually in the United States. The average lifetime is only a little more than forty years. It should be at least one hundred years. This is a very conservative statement, for many live to be considerably older, and it is within the power of each individual to prolong his life beyond what is now considered old age.

Under favorable conditions people should live in comfort and health to the age of one hundred years or more, useful and in full possession of their faculties. Barring accidents, which should be less numerous when people fully realize that unreasonable haste and speed are wasteful and that life is more valuable than accumulated wealth, human life could and should be a certainty. There should be no sudden deaths resulting from the popular diseases of today. In fact, pneumonia, typhoid fever, tuberculosis, cancer and various other ills that are fatal to the vast majority of the race, should and could be abolished. This may sound idealistic, but though such results are not probable in the near future, they are possible.

All civilized nations of which we have record, except the Chinese, have decayed after growing and flourishing a few centuries, usually about a thousand years or less. Many reasons are given for the decline and fall of nations. Rome especially furnishes food for much thought. However, look into the history of each known nation that has risen to prominence, glory and power, and you will find that so long as they kept in close contact with the soil they flourished. With the advance of civilization the peoples change their mode of life from simplicity to luxuriousness and complexity. Thus individuals decay and in the end there is enough individual decay to result in national degeneration. When this process has advanced far enough these people are unable to hold their own. In the severe competitition of nations the strain is too great and they perish. There is a point of refinement beyond which people can not go and survive.

From luxury nations are plunged into hardship. Then their renewed contact with the soil gradually causes their regeneration, if they have enough vitality left to rise again. Such is the history of the Italians. Many others, like the once great Egyptians, whose civilization was very far advanced and who became so dissolute that a virtuous woman was a curiosity, have been unable to recover, even after a lapse of many centuries. The degenerated nations are like diseased individuals: Some have gone so far on the road to ruin that they are doomed to die. Others can slowly regain their health by mending their ways.

Nations, like individuals, generally do better in moderate circumstances than in opulence. Nearly all can stand poverty, but only the exceptional individual or nation can bear up under riches. Nature demands of us that we exercise both body and mind.

Civilization is not inimical to health and long life. In fact, the contrary is true, for as the people advance they learn to master the forces of nature and with these forces under control they are able to lead better, healthier lives, but if they become too soft and luxurious there is decay of moral and physical fibre, and in the end the nation must fall, for its individual units are unworthy of survival in a world which requires an admixture of brain and brawn.

Civilization is favorable to long life so long as the people are moderate and live simply, but when it degenerates to sensuous softness, individual and racial deterioration ensue. Among savages the infant mortality is very great, but such ills as cancer, tuberculosis, smallpox and Bright's disease are rare. These are luxuries which are generally introduced with civilization. Close housing, too generous supply of food, too little exercise and alcohol are some of the fatal blessings which civilized man introduces among savages.

A part of the price we must pay for being civilized is the exercise of considerable self-control and self-denial, otherwise we must suffer.

The state of the individual health is not satisfactory. There is too much illness, too much suffering and too many premature deaths. It is estimated that in our country about three millions of people are ill each day, on the average. The monetary loss is tremendous and the anguish and suffering are beyond estimate.

The race is losing every year a vast army of individuals who are in their productive prime. When a part of a great city is destroyed men give careful consideration to the material loss and plan to prevent a recurrence. But that is nothing compared to the loss we suffer from the annual death of a host of experienced men and women. Destroyed business blocks can be replaced, but it is impossible to replace men and women.

We look upon this unnecessary waste of life complacently because we are used to it and consequently think that it is natural. It is neither necessary nor natural. If we would read and heed nature's writings it would cease. Then people would live until their time came to fade away peacefully and beautifully, as do the golden leaves of autumn or the blades of grass.

Many dread old age because they think of it in connection with decrepitude, helplessness and the childish querulousness popularly associated with advancing years. This is not a natural old age; it is disease. Natural old age is sweet, tolerant and cheerful. There are few things in life more precious than the memory of parents and grandparents grown old gracefully, after having weathered the storms of appetites and passions, the mind firmly enthroned and filled with the calm toleration and wisdom that come with the passing years of a well spent life.

A busy mind in a healthy body does not degenerate. The brain, though apparently unstable, is one of the most stable parts of the body.

We should desire and acquire health because when healthy we are at our maximum efficiency. We are able to enjoy life. We have greater capacity for getting and giving. We live more fully. Being normal, we are in harmony with ourselves and with our associates. We are of greater value all around. We are better citizens.

Every individual owes something to the race. It is our duty to contribute our part so that the result of our lives is not a tendency toward degeneration, but toward upbuilding, of the race. The part played by each individual is small, but the aggregate is great. If our children are better born and better brought up than we were, and there is generally room for improvement, we have at least helped.

Health is within the grasp of all who are not afflicted with organic disease, and the vast majority have no organic ills. All that is necessary is to lead natural lives and learn how to use the mind properly. Those who are not in sympathy with the views on racial duty can enhance their personal worth through better living without giving the race any thought. Every individual who leads a natural life and thinks to advantage helps to bring about better public health. The national health is the aggregate of individual health and is improved as the individuals evolve into better health. National or racial improvement come through evolution, not through revolution. The improvement is due to small contributions from many sources.

The greatest power for human uplift is knowledge. Reformers often believe that they can improve the world by legislation. Lasting reform comes through education. If the laws are very repressive the reaction is both great and unpleasant.

It takes about six months to learn stenography. It requires a long apprenticeship to become a first-class blacksmith or horseshoer. To obtain the rudiments of a physician's art it is necessary to spend four to six years in college. To learn a language takes an apt pupil at least a year. A lawyer must study from two to four years to become a novice. A businessman must work many years before he is an expert in his line. Not one of these attainments is worth as much as good health, yet an individual of average intelligence can obtain enough knowledge about right living during his spare time in from two to six months to assure him of good health, if he lives as well as he knows how. Is it worth while? It certainly is, for it is one of the essentials of life. Health will increase one's earning capacity and productivity and more than double both the pleasure and the duration of life.

Disease is a very expensive luxury. Health is one of the cheapest, though one of the rarest, things on earth. There is no royal road to health. If there is any law of health it is this: Only those will retain it permanently who are deserving of it.

Many prefer to live in that state of uncertainty, which may be called tolerable health, a state in which they do not suffer, yet are not quite well. In this condition they have their little ups and downs and occasionally a serious illness, which too often proves fatal. Even such people ought to acquire health knowledge, for the time may come when they will desire to enjoy life to the fullest, which they can do only when they have health. Those who have this knowledge are often able to help themselves quickly and effectively when no one else can.

I am acquainted with many who have been educated out of disease into health. Many of them are indiscreet, but they have learned to know the signs of approaching trouble and they ease up before anything serious overtakes them. In this way they save themselves and their families from much suffering, much anxiety and much expense. Every adult should know enough to remain well. Every one should know the signs of approaching illness and how to abort it. The mental comfort and ease that come from the possession of such knowledge are priceless.

Everything that is worth while must be paid for in some way and the price of continued good health is some basic knowledge and self-control. There are no hardships connected with rational living. It means to live moderately and somewhat more simply than is customary. Simplicity reduces the amount of work and friction and adds to the enjoyment of life. The cheerfulness, the buoyancy and the tingling with the joy of life that come to those who have perfect health more than compensate for the pet bad habits which must be given up.

Many of the popular teachings regarding disease and its prevention are false. The germ theory is a delusion. The fact will some day be generally recognized, as it is today by a few, that the so-called pathogenic bacteria or germs have no power to injure a healthy body, that there is bodily degeneration first and then the system becomes a favorable culture medium for germs: In other words, disease comes first and the pathogenic bacteria multiply afterwards. This view may seem very ridiculous to the majority, for it is a strong tenet of popular medical belief today that micro-organisms are the cause of most diseases.

To most people, medical and lay, the various diseases stand out clear and individual. Typhoid fever is one disease. Pneumonia is an entirely different one. Surely this is so, they say, for is not typhoid fever due to the bacillus typhosus and pneumonia to the pneumococcus? But it is not so. Outside of mechanical injuries there is but one disease, and the various conditions that we dignify with individual names are but manifestations of this disease. The parent disease is filthiness, and its manifestations vary according to circumstances and individuals.

This filthiness is not of the skin, but of the interior of the body. The blood stream becomes unclean, principally because of indigestion and constipation, which are chiefly due to improper eating habits. Some of the contributory causes are wrong thinking, too little exercise, lack of fresh air, and ingestion of sedatives and stimulants which upset the assimilative and excretory functions of the body. In all cases the blood is unclean. The patient is suffering from autointoxication or autotoxemia.

If this is true, it would follow that the treatment of all diseases is about the same. For instance, it would be necessary to give about the same treatment for eczema as for pneumonia. Basically, that is exactly what has to be done to obtain the best results, though the variation in location and manifestation requires that special relief measures, of lesser importance, be used in special cases, to get the quickest and best results. In both eczema and pneumonia the essential thing is to get the body clean.

The practice of medicine is not a science. We have drugs that are reputed to be excellent healers, yet these very drugs sometimes produce death within a few hours of being taken. The practice of medicine is an art, and the outcome in various cases depends more on the personality of the artist than on the drugs he gives, for roughly speaking, all medicines are either sedative or stimulant, and if the dosage is kept below the danger line, the patient generally recovers. It seems to make very little difference whether the medicine is given in the tiny homeopathic doses, so small that they have only a suggestive effect, or if they are given in doses several hundred times as large by allopaths and eclectics.

It is true that we have drugs with which we can diminish or increase the number of heart beats per minute, dilate or contract the pupils of the eye, check or stimulate the secretion of mucus, sedate or irritate the nervous system, etc., but all that is accomplished is temporary stimulation or sedation, and such juggling does not cure. The practice of medicine is today what it has been in the past, largely experiment and guess-work.

On the other hand, natural healers who have drunk deep of the cup of knowledge need not guess. They know that withholding of food and cleaning out the alimentary tract will reduce a fever. They know that the same measures will clean up foul wounds and stop the discharge of pus in a short time. They know that the same measures in connection with hot baths will terminate headaches and remove pain. They further know that if the patient will take the proper care of himself after the acute manifestations have disappeared there will be no more disease. After a little experience, an intelligent natural healer can tell his patients, in the majority of cases, what to expect if instructions are followed. He can say positively that there will be no relapses and no complications.

How different is this from the unsatisfactory practice of conventional medicine! However, most physicians refuse to accept the valuable teachings which are offered to them freely, and one of the reasons is that the natural healers do not present their knowledge in scientific form. The knowledge is scientific but it is simple. Such objection does not come with good grace from a profession practicing an art. Life is but a tiny part science, mixed with much art.

The true scientist in the healing art is he who can take an invalid and by the use of the means at his command bring him back to health, not in an accidental manner, but in such a knowing way that he can predict the outcome. In serious cases the natural healer of intelligence and experience can do this twenty times where the man who relies on drugs does it once. The physicians who prescribe drugs are ever on the look-out for complications and relapses, and they have many of them. The natural healers know that under proper treatment neither complications nor relapses can occur, unless the disease has already advanced so far that the vital powers are exhausted before treatment is begun, and this is generally not the case. In this book many of the medical fallacies of today, both professional and lay, will be touched upon in a kindly spirit of helpfulness and ideas that contain more truth will be offered in their place. The truth is the best knowledge we have today, according to our understanding. It is not fixed, for it may be replaced by something better tomorrow. However, one fundamental truth regarding health will never change, namely, that it is necessary to conform to the laws of nature, or in other words, the laws of our being, in order to retain it.

No one can cover the field of health completely, for though it is very simple, it is as big as life. The most helpful parts of this book will be those which point the way for each individual to understand his relation to what we call nature, and hence help to enable him to gain a better understanding of himself.

By natural living is not meant the discarding of the graces of civilization and roaming about in adamic costume, living on the foods as they are found in forest and field, without preparation. What is meant is the adjustment of each person to his environment, or the environment to the person, until harmony or balance is established, which means health.

One of the most difficult things about teaching health is that it is so very simple. People look for something mysterious. When told that good old mother nature is the only healer, they are incredulous, for they have been taught that doctors cure. When informed that they do not need medicine and that outside treatment is unnecessary, they find it difficult to believe, for disease has always called for treatment of some kind in the hands of the medical profession. When further told that they have to help themselves by living so that they will not put any obstacles in the way of normal functioning of their bodies, they think that the physician who thinks and talks that way must be a crank, and many seek help where they are told that they can obtain health from pills, powders and potions or from various inoculations and injections.

To live in health is so simple that any intelligent person can master the art and furthermore regain lost health in the average case, without any help from professional healers. There is plenty knowledge and all that is needed is a discriminating mind to find the truth and then exercise enough will power to live it. If a good healer is at hand, it is cheaper to pay his fee for personal advice than to try to evolve into health without aid, but if it is a burden to pay the price, get the knowledge and practice it and health will return in most cases. The vast majority of people suffering from chronic ills which are considered incurable can get well by living properly.

The more capable and frank the healer is, the less treatment will be administered. Minute examinations and frequent treatment serve to make the patient believe that he is getting a great deal for his money. Advice is what the healer has to sell, and if it is correct, it is precious. The patient should not object to paying a reasonable fee, for what he learns is good for life. People gladly pay for prescriptions or drugs. The latter are injurious if taken in sufficient quantity to have great effect. So why object to paying for health education, which is more valuable than all the drugs in the world? Because of their attitude on this subject, the people force many a doctor to use drugs, who would gladly practice in a more reasonable way if it would bring the necessities of life to him and his family. The public has to enlighten itself before it will get good health advice. The medical men will continue in the future, as they have done in the past, to furnish the kind of service that is popular.

A good natural healer teaches his patients to get along without him and other doctors. A doctor of the conventional school teaches his patrons to depend upon him. The former is consequently deserving of far greater reward than the latter.

The law of compensation may apply elsewhere, thinks the patient, but surely it is nonsense to teach that it applies in matters of health, for does not everybody know that most of our diseases are due to causes over which we have no control? That the chief cause is germs and that we can not control the air well enough to prevent one of these horrible monsters (about 1/25,000 of an inch long) from settling in the body and multiplying, at last producing disease and maybe death? This is untrue, but it is a very comforting theory, for it removes the element of personal responsibility. People do not like to be told that if they are ill it is their own fault, that they are only reaping as they have sowed, yet such is the truth.

Patients often dislike to give up one or more of their bad habits. "Mr. Blank has done this very thing for sixty or seventy years and now at the age of eighty or ninety he is strong and active," they reply to warnings. This is sophistry, for although an individual occasionally lives to old age in spite of broken health laws, the average person who attempts it perishes young. Those who do not conform to the rules are not allowed to sit in the game to the end.

Another false feeling, or rather hope, deeply implanted in the human breast is: "Perhaps others can not do this, but I can. I have done it before and can do it again; it will not hurt me for I am strong and possessed of a good constitution." The wish is father to the thought, which is not founded on facts. The most common and the most destructive form of dishonesty is self-deception. Those who are honest with themselves find it easy to deal fairly and squarely with others.

The doctors of the dominant school are very distrustful of the natural healers, in spite of the fact that the latter obtain the best results. Many of the conditions which the regular physicians treat without satisfactory results, the natural healers are able to remove in a few months. When members of the dominant school of medicine find men leading patients suffering from various skin diseases, Bright's disease, chronic digestive troubles, rheumatism and other ills which they themselves make little or no impression upon back to health, they are unwilling to believe that such results can be accomplished by means of hygiene and proper feeding. They think there is some fakery about it, for their professors, books and experience have taught them otherwise. They consider the views of the natural healer unworthy of serious attention and often call him a quack, which epithet closes the discussion. They are ethical and do not wish to be mired by contact with quacks.

The distrust of medical men for healers of the natural school is not hard to explain. Many of the natural healers are men of education and experience, but others lack both, and no matter how good the latter may be at heart, they make very serious blunders. For instance: They get out circulars, listing all prominent diseases known, stating that they cure them. They either are so enthusiastic that they are carried away or they are so ignorant that they do not know that there is a stage of degeneration which will not allow of regeneration, and that when such a stage is reached in any chronic disease the end is death.

Another handicap is that intelligent natural healers have such excellent success that they lose their heads. They educate patients by the hundred into health who have been given up as incurable by the conventional physicians. In their success they forget that modesty is very becoming to the successful and begin to boast. This hurts the cause. Let the natural healer ever remember that he does not cure, that he is but the interpreter and that nature is the restorer of health.

The natural healers must be more careful about their statements if they would have the respect of intelligent people, and they must labor diligently to be well informed. For their own good regular physicians will have to be more open-minded, and recognize the fact that it is not necessary to have a M. D. degree to accept the truth regarding healing. Medical men are losing their hold on the public largely because they have cultivated the class spirit.

It is a well known fact among natural healers that most cases of Bright's disease are curable, even after they have become chronic. However, a physician who voices this truth will probably be classed among irresponsible dreamers by other doctors.

Antagonism of this kind breeds extremists and is therefore harmful to the public, which pays for all the mistakes made. It is very easy to lose one's mental balance and to begin to play on a harp with but one string. We have a large army of Christian Scientists. If it were not for the way in which physicians of the past mistreated the body and neglected the mind, this sect would not exist. The doctors, with their awful doses of nauseous and destructive drugs, went to one extreme. The reaction was the formation of a sect that has gone to the other extreme. The Christian Scientists are incomprehensible in spots to us mortals who believe in a body as well as a mind, but they have a cheerful and helpful philosophy which brings enjoyment on earth and they have done an immense amount of good by teaching people to cease thinking and talking so much about themselves and their ills. Among other demonstrations, they have shown the uselessness of drugs.

Of late so many varieties of drugless healers have sprung into existence that it is difficult to remember even their names. There are many pathies. These have a tendency to take one part of the human being, or one procedure of treatment, and to play this up to the elimination of all the rest. Some do everything with the mind. Others pay no attention to the mind. Bathing, massage, manipulating the spine, washing out the colon, baths in mud, sunshine or water, suggestion and many other things are separately given credit for being cure-alls. Many of these are excellent as a part of regenerative treatment, but they are not sufficient of themselves to give permanent results.

Most healers have too narrow vision. People come to them because they have faith. The faith alone will produce temporary improvement, but as soon as the interest is gone and the procedure grows old the patient becomes worse again unless the treatment possesses genuine merit. Osteopathy is most excellent, as a part of a healing system, but it is not sufficient. The osteopaths find their patients relapsing over and over again, or taking some other disease. However, they are learning, in increasing numbers, that if they would keep their patrons well, they have to give them education along the line of hygiene and dietetics, with a little mental training thrown in.

Many chiropractors are learning the same thing. In some chiropractic schools there are professors wise enough to teach their students to be broad-minded. The true natural healer makes use of air, water, food, exercise, mental training--in fact, all the means nature has put at his disposal. He realizes that the best treatment is education of the patient. In many cases a cure can be greatly hastened by proper local treatment.

It is unfortunate that the nature healers are so divided and that many operate upon such a narrow basis. If the vast majority of them were well informed, broad enough to make use of all helpful natural means, and were designated by the same name, it would not take them long to gain more public confidence and respect than they now possess. So long as the nature healers segregate themselves and allow themselves to be narrow, so long will they have to struggle at a disadvantage against the more united wielders of scalpels and prescribers of drugs.

The question of choosing a health guide is sometimes perplexing. The patient should select one in whom he has confidence, for confidence is a great aid in restoring health. It often happens that there is no one in the town in whom the patient has confidence, for many communities have no competent natural healers. Then the question is whether or not to seek advice by correspondence. In acute diseases this is generally a bad plan, for the family often lacks the poise and equanimity necessary to carry out directions. In chronic cases it is usually all right. Here all that is required is correct knowledge put into practice and errors are not as dangerous as in acute diseases. Curable cases will get well by following the advice given by correspondence. A medical man who educates people by correspondence is considered unethical and is severely censured by the ethical brethren. To prescribe medicine by mail is without doubt reprehensible, but to educate people into health is a work of merit, whether it is done face to face or by correspondence. It is advantageous to meet the physician, talk things over and be examined, but it is not necessary.

I know of some cases of acute disease treated satisfactorily by letter and telegram, but the patients' families were in sympathy with natural methods, of which they had a fair knowledge, and they had unlimited confidence in the healer.

I am personally acquainted with many people who have been educated out of chronic disease and into health by correspondence, after the local physicians had vainly exhausted all their skill. It is simply a matter of applied knowledge and it works just as well in curable cases if given by telephone, telegraph or letter as if imparted by word of mouth. However, it seems to me that it is most satisfactory for all concerned when the healer and the sufferer can meet.

My words are not inspired by any ill feeling toward the members of the medical profession. I have found medical men to measure well up in every way. They are better educated than the average and they are as kind and considerate as are other men. As men we can expect no more of them under present conditions, but because they are better equipped than the average, we have a right to ask for an improvement in their practice, even if they have inherited a great many handicaps from their predecessors and it is not easy to throw off the past, which acts as a dead weight ever tending to check progress. The tendency of the times is for fuller, freer and more sincere service in every line, for evolving out of the useless into the greatest helpfulness. It is not asking too much when we demand of the doctors that they rid themselves of the injurious drug superstition and become health teachers, that instead of being in the rear they come to the front and make progress easier.

What I say about drugs is founded on intimate observation. I was educated medically in two of the colleges where medication is strongly advocated and well taught, and am a regular M. D. I have watched people who were treated by means of drugs and the biologic products, such as serums, vaccines and bacterines, which are now so popular, and I have watched many who have been treated by natural methods. Anyone with my experience and capable of thinking would come to the conclusions given in this book, that it is a mistake to administer drugs and serums and that the natural methods give results so much superior to the conventional methods that there is no comparison. Others who have discarded drugs know from experience that this is true.

The physicians who are on intimate terms with nature will neither desire nor require drugs. Sound advice, that is, teaching, is the most valuable service a physician can render. Right living and right thinking always result in health if no serious organic degeneration has taken place. If the public could only be made to realize that they need a great deal of knowledge and very little treatment, and that knowledge is very valuable and treatment often worthless the day would soon dawn when health matters will be placed on a sound, natural basis.

Surgery is occasionally necessary, but today from ten to twenty operations are performed where but one is needed.

"There is nothing new beneath the sun," is a popular quotation. It seems to hold true in the healing art, for the best modern practice was the best ancient practice. Naturally, people like to make new discoveries and get credit therefore. Our valuable new discoveries in healing are very ancient. Though much that appears in these pages may seem strange and new to many, I claim no originality. My aim is to present workable, helpful facts in such a way that any person of average intelligence and will power can apply them, and to get the essentials of health within such a compass that no unreasonable amount of time need be employed in finding them.

According to late discoveries, the ancient Egyptians were more advanced in the art of living than any other people on earth, including the moderns. They taught that overeating is the chief causative factor of disease, and so it is. They taught cleanliness, the priests going to the extreme of shaving the entire body daily. It would naturally follow that they prescribed moderation in eating, which leads to internal cleanliness. Cleanliness of body, in conjunction with cleanliness of mind, will put disease to rout.

The ancient Greek writers commented on the good state of health among the Egyptians, and modern medical writers marvel that they made so little use of drugs. Evidently they found drugs of little value, for they were taught hygienic living. The admirable health laws laid down by Moses were derived from Egyptian sources.

The ancient nations were as much influenced by the Egyptians as we are today by the Greeks who lived before the Christian era. The Greeks built combination temples and sanitaria, to which the afflicted resorted. The priests were in charge and these ancient heathens were great rogues. By fooling the people they got big fees out of them. Their oracular sayings and miracles were adroitly presented. They did not teach that overeating is the chief cause of disease, for this did not suit the mystic times. The people liked oracular prescriptions, and they got them. The law of supply and demand worked as well then as it does now. The heathen priests waxed fat and the medical art degenerated.

About five centuries B. C., Pythagoras taught that health can be preserved by means of proper diet, exercise and the right use of the mind. He also taught many other truths and some fallacies. In spite of much superstition mixed with his philosophy, it was too pure for the times and he perished.

Hippocrates, born about 470 years B. C., is one of the bright lights of the medical world. He was so far ahead of his time that he still lives. He was the founder of medical art as we know it. He used many drugs, but he also relied on natural means. He was the first medical man on record to pay serious attention to dietetics. The following quotations will show how well his mind grasped the essentials of the healing art: "Old persons need less fuel (food) than the young." "In winter abundant nourishment is wholesome; in summer a more frugal diet." "Follow nature." "Complete abstinence often acts very well, if the strength of the patient can in any way maintain it." In acute disease he withheld nourishment at first and then he prescribed a liquid diet. He also made use of the "milk cure," which is considered modern, in conjunction with baths and exercise; this is very efficacious in some chronic diseases. He further spoke the oft-forgotten truth that physicians do not heal. "Natural powers are the healers of disease." "Nature suffices for everything under all conditions."

The next great physician was Galen, who lived in the second and third centuries of our era. He added greatly to medical knowledge, made extensive use of dietetics, and then in a self-satisfied manner informed his readers that they need look no further for enlightenment, for he had given them all that was of any value. Perhaps he meant this as a joke, but those who followed him took it seriously, with the result that medical advance stopped for several centuries.

The physicians of the dark ages had some light, as evidenced by this popular quotation taken from a poem that the faculty of the medical college of Salerno gave to Robert, son of William the Conqueror, in the year 1101:

"Salerno's school in conclave high unites To counsel England's king and thus indites: If thou to health and vigor wouldst attain, Shun mighty cares, all anger deem profane; From heavy suppers and much wine abstain; Nor trivial count it after pompous fare To rise from table and to take the air. Shun idle noonday slumbers, nor delay The urgent calls of nature to obey. These rules if thou wilt follow to the end, Thy life to greater length thou may'st extend."

During recent times but two important discoveries have been made concerning matters of health: First, the advantage of cleanliness; second, the approximate chemical composition of various foods. All the other important new discoveries are old.

Cleanliness, moderation in all things, right thinking and a realization of the fact that nature cures are some of the most important stones upon which to build a healing practice. The most important single therapeutic factor is to abstain from food during pain and active disease processes.

Cleanliness of mind and body has been taught for thousands of years, yet cleanliness of body is a new discovery, for which we are greatly indebted to the great bacteriologist, Pasteur. It has been found that germs thrive best in filth; this has been taught so thoroughly that the public is somewhat afraid of the germs and as a measure of self-protection they are cleaning up. Of old, cleanliness meant a clean skin, but this is the least important part. It is far more necessary to have a clean alimentary tract and clean blood, with a resultant sweet, healthy body, and this is what cleanliness is beginning to mean. Internal cleanliness necessitates moderation, for an overworked alimentary tract becomes foul and some of the poisons are taken into the blood.

Asepsis and antisepsis simply mean cleanliness.

The benefits of moderation have been known for thousands of years. Louis Cornaro, who died in 1566, wrote a delightful book on the subject. People know that it is necessary to be moderate, but they do not seem to realize the meaning of moderation nor is its value well enough implanted in the human mind to produce satisfactory results.

Right thinking seemed as important to the thinkers of old as it does to the New Thought people today. "As a man thinketh in his heart, so is he."

For the better knowledge of the composition of food we have to thank the chemists.

Laymen are referred to frequently in this book because their work has been so helpful and important. Herbert Spencer and Alfred Russel Wallace had very clear conceptions regarding health. See their opinions regarding vaccination. There is no difference in the mental processes of physicians and laymen. Anyone can know about health, though it takes considerable experience and observation to get acquainted with the less important subject of disease. One indictment against medical men is that they have dwelled almost entirely on disease and paid no attention to health.

A group of modern men deserve great credit for popularizing health knowledge, which generally results in the loss of professional standing of the teacher. R. H. Trall, M. D., insisted that drugs are useless and harmful, that the only rational and safe way of healing ordinary ills is to use nature's means. "Strictly speaking, fever and food are antagonistic ideas," he wrote. In his Hydropathic Encyclopedia, copyrighted in 1851, he puts great stress on natural remedies, such as food and water. He met with much opposition, but he has left a deep impression on the minds of men who are now having some influence in shaping public opinion on health and healing.

Dr. Charles Page of Boston has been writing in advocacy of natural healing for over thirty years. He also has emphasized the harmfulness of drugs, the necessity of withholding food from fever patients, and simple living, remaining in touch with nature. Another important point which the doctor has been trying to impress upon the public is that it is necessary to retain the natural salts of the foods, instead of ruining them or throwing them away, as is generally done, especially in the preparation of vegetables and many cereal products.

Dr. Edward Hooker Dewey began to present his ideas to the public a few years after the Civil War. His little book entitled "The No-Breakfast Plan and the Fasting Cure," has had a great influence among rational healers. The doctor emphasized the importance of going without food in acute diseases so that no one who has read the book can forget it. He pointed out some of the errors of conventional healing as they had never been shown before, and I believe he was the first one to give the correct rules to guide people in the consumption of food.

For fourteen years Dr. J. H. Tilden of Denver has been a voluminous writer on health. He teaches that the law of compensation applies to health; that all disease is one and the same fundamentally; that "Autotoxemia is the fundamental basic cause of all diseases." Like all others who have investigated the subject impartially he believes that one of the most important factors of health is correct feeding. He allows all foods, in compatible combinations. Of course, he gives no drugs.

Dr. Harry Brook of Los Angeles is unique among the health educators of today. He is a brainy journalist with a good stock of fundamental health knowledge and is endowed with the ability to place his convictions before the public in a striking manner. He has been carrying on his educational work for many years.

Elbert Hubbard has also had a great deal of influence on the thought of today. At intervals he publishes an article on health which gets wide distribution. He has the faculty of making people think, and those who allow themselves to think independently generally evolve into serviceable knowledge.

Bernarr Macfadden has a large following. He is a strong advocate of physical culture and favors vegetarianism and other changes from conventional life. He educates his readers away from drugs. He has written much that is helpful and his influence is widely felt. Like all others who have struggled against the fetters of convention, he has aroused much opposition.

There are a few good health magazines, and there are many people living who deserve credit for their labor to improve the mental and physical condition of humanity. Some of these will be mentioned and quoted.

Some of the teachers have dwelled upon but one idea and some have advocated fallacies, but there is good to be found in all of them. No knowledge assays one hundred per cent. pure.

No helpful healing knowledge should be kept away from the public; it should be as free as possible. The public, when it understands, willingly pays a fair price for it, which is all that should be asked. To take advantage of the sick and helpless is contemptible. The old-time idea, still prevalent, that medical knowledge is for the doctor only is a mistake. The best patients are the intelligent ones. The office of the physician should be to educate his clients; his best knowledge and his best qualities will be developed in dealing honestly with intelligent people.

The practice of medical secrecy began in ancient times when the healers and the priests believed in fooling the public. Unfortunately, this professional attitude still survives. No one who has not practiced the healing art can know how tempted a doctor is to fake and humbug a little to retain and gain patronage.

Emerson wrote: "He is the rich man who can avail himself of other men's faculties. He is the richest man who knows how to draw a benefit from the labors of the greatest number of men--of men in distant countries and past times." Those who wish to be healthy and efficient are compelled to advance by taking advantage of other men's faculties. He who attempts to learn all by experience does not live long enough to travel far.

Everyone should try to get a knowledge of the few most fundamental facts of nature governing life. Then it would not be so easy to go astray. Health literature should be read with an open mind. Read in conjunction with your knowledge of the laws of nature, and then it will be seen that health and disease are according to law, and that by eliminating the mistakes disease will disappear.

All disease is one. It is the manifestation of disobeyed natural law, and whether the mistakes are made knowingly or ignorantly matters but little so far as the results are concerned. It is generally considered a disgrace to be imprisoned for transgressing man-made law, which is faulty and complex. How about being in the fetters of disease for disregarding nature's law, which is just and simple?

It is my aim to use as simple language as possible. If physicians read these pages, they will understand them without technicalities, and so will laymen. This book contains much knowledge that physicians should have, knowledge that will help them when that which they have acquired from conventional sources fails, but in many respects it is so opposed to popular customs and beliefs that many physicians will doubtless condemn it on first reading. Doctors are taught otherwise at medical colleges, and most of them have such high regard for authority that it is very difficult for them to see matters in a different light. I appeal to both laymen and healers with open minds.

These rambling thoughts will serve to show the reader whether it is worth while to go any further. The following chapters are devoted to an exposition of a workable knowledge of how to retain health, and how to regain lost health in ordinary cases. They will teach how to get dependable health, how to remain well in spite of climatic conditions, bacteria and other factors that are given as causes of disease, and how to more than double the ordinary span of life.

Good health and long life result in better work, increased earning capacity and efficiency of body and mind, greater understanding, and more enjoyment of life. It gives time to cultivate wisdom.

CHAPTER II.

MENTAL ATTITUDE.

On mental questions there is a wide divergence of opinion. At one extreme some say that all is mind, at the other, that life is entirely physical, that the mind is but a refined part of the body. Most of us recognize both body and mind, and realize that life has a physical basis. If some are pleased to be known as mental phenomena, no harm is done.

All desire to make a success of life. What would be a success for one would be a failure for another. It all depends on the point of view. Broadly speaking, all are successful who are helpful, whether it be in furnishing pleasure or necessities to others. The humble may be as successful as the great, yes even more so.

Wealth and success are not synonymous, as many think. Among the failures must be counted many of the wealthy. Financial success is not real success unless it has been gained in return for valuable service. The men of initiative deserve greater rewards than the plodders and these rewards are cheerfully given.

A little genuine love and affection can bring more beauty and happiness into life than wealth, and neither can be bought with money.

The best and most satisfying form of success comes to him who helps himself by helping others. "It is more blessed to give than to receive," has passed into common currency; but the more we give the more we receive. He who loves attracts love. He who hates is repaid in kind. "He who lives by the sword shall perish by the sword."

The enjoyment of the fruits of one's labor is a part of success. Some make a fetish of success and thus lose out. Others are so ambitious that in their striving they forget to live. A little ambition is good; too much sows the seed of struggle, strife and discontent and defeats its own ends. Those who do evil because the end justifies the means have already buried some of the best that is in them.

To enjoy life, health of body and mind is necessary. The mind can not come to full fruitage without a good body. Those who strive so hard to reach a certain goal that they neglect the physical become wrecks and after a few years of discomfort and disease are consigned to premature graves. Through proper living and thinking the body and mind are built up, not only enough to meet ordinary demands upon them, but extraordinary ones. In other words, it is within our power to have a large margin, balance or reserve of physical and mental force.

To make the meaning clearer let us illustrate financially: Prudent people lay aside a few dollars from time to time, in a savings bank, for instance. All goes well and the savings grow. At last there are one thousand dollars. Now an emergency arises, and if the saver can not furnish nine hundred dollars he will lose his home. In this case he must either borrow or use his reserve, so he takes nine hundred dollars from the savings bank and keeps his home. The improvident man loses his home under similar circumstances, for his credit is not good and he has no balance to draw upon.

And it is the same with physical and mental powers, except that we can not borrow these, no matter how much good will or credit we may have. He who lives well is accumulating a reserve. He has a wide margin. If trouble comes he can draw upon his reserve energy or surplus resistance and bridge it over. He may be tired out, but he escapes with body and mind intact.

The imprudent liver generally has such a narrow margin that any extraordinary demand made upon him breaks him down. It is very common for men to die after a financial failure. Disease, insanity and death often follow family trouble or the loss of a dear one. The reason is that such people live up to their limit every day. They have no margin to work on. They either overdo or underdo and fail to become balanced. Then a little physical or mental exertion beyond the ordinary often means a breakage or extinction.

Equanimity and moderation will help to build up the reserve and give the resistance that is necessary to cope successfully with the unforeseen difficulties that we sometimes have to surmount.

The physical state depends largely on the mental state and vice versa. Body and mind react upon each other. Bad blood does not only cause abnormal functioning of such organs as the heart, liver, kidneys and lungs, but it interferes with the normal functioning of the brain. It diminishes the mental output and causes a deterioration of the quality. An engorged liver makes a man cranky. Indigestion causes pessimism. Physical pain is so disturbing that the sufferer thinks mostly of himself and is unable to perform his work well. We never do our best when self-conscious. If there is severe pain the mind can perform no useful labor.

On the other hand, anger stops digestion and poisons the secretions of the body. Worry does the same. It takes the mind from constructive thoughts and deeds and centers it upon ourselves. An effective mind must be tranquil, otherwise it upsets the body and fails to give proper direction to our activities.

For a real life success we need a proper perspective. We need to be balanced, poised, adjusted. Most of us are too circumscribed mentally. We live so much by and for ourselves that we consider ourselves, individually, of greater importance than the facts warrant. Others do not agree with us on this point, and this is a source of disturbance. I am personally acquainted with two surgeons and several physicians who think they are the greatest in the world, and one considers himself the best physician of all time. The rest of the world does not appraise them so highly, and some of these professional men are very much annoyed because of this lack of appreciation.

Selfishness and self-esteem to a certain point are virtues. Beyond that point they become vices. Certainly we should think well of ourselves, and then act so that this good opinion is merited. Self-interest and selfishness are the main-springs of progress. Most of us need some inducement to do good work. It is well that it is so. The ones who deserve the great rewards generally get them, whether they are mental or physical.

To obtain a proper perspective of ourselves we must learn to think independently and honestly. It is too common to be conventionally honest, but dishonest with ourselves. It is too common to pass unnoticed in ourselves the faults we condemn in others. We should be lenient in our judgment because often the mistakes that others make would have been ours had we but had the opportunity to make them.

As physical ills are principally caused by bad physical habits, so are mental ills and inefficiency chiefly due to various bad mental habits, which are allowed to fasten themselves upon us. These will be briefly discussed so as to focus attention upon them, for the first thing necessary for the correction of a bad habit is to recognize its presence. It is as important to think right as it is to give the body proper care. A good body with a mind working in the wrong direction is of no use. If we allow our minds to be disturbed and distressed by every little unfavorable happening, we shall never have enough tranquility to think well.

The proper time to quit our bad habits is now. Why wait until the first of the month or the first of the year? Every day that we harbor a bad habit it grows greater and strikes deeper and stronger roots. A child one year old can often be broken of a bad habit in a week; a child of three, within a month; a child of six, within a few months; but let the habit grow until the age of twenty, and it may take a year or more to break the bonds. Let it continue until the age of thirty, and the victim will say, "I can quit any time," but the chances are that the habit will remain for life. After the individual is fifty or sixty years old, he is rarely capable of changing. If he is the victim of a very bad habit, it has generally so sapped his strength of body and mind that he is unable to break away.

The right time to stop bad habits is now.

Some people have many pet bad habits. It is often the best policy to attack them one at a time. Those who try to conquer all at once often fail. They backslide, lose self-confidence, become discouraged, tell themselves that it is no use, for it can not be done. Begin with the habit that is least formidable. After this is conquered, overcome another one, and in time most of the bad habits will be subdued. The first conquest builds confidence, and with confidence and determination it is possible to gain self-mastery in time.

The greatest evil about bad habits is that they conquer us. They become masters, we slaves. Let us be free. "He who conquers himself is greater than he who taketh a city."

The mind grows strong by overcoming obstacles, as the body gains in strength through work and exercise.

Giving up bad habits is very disagreeable at first. Those who have conquered the prevalent habit of overeating know that they have been in a fight. The smokers who quit suffer. Those who break away from liquor have a much greater struggle. Those who attempt to overcome drug addictions suffer the tortures of the damned. Those who overcome their bad mental habits have a hard time of it at first, but though it is difficult it is possible. It is no easy matter to curb a fiery disposition or to quit worrying. It requires time, persistence and perseverance. Fretting, envy, spite, jealousy and hatred are tenacious tenants of the mind they occupy. These harmful emotions are enemies which sap our strength and we must thrust them from our lives if we would live well. This is not all narrow selfishness, for when we have gained mental calm for ourselves we are in position to impart peace of mind to others and to be more useful than previously. A calm mind is not a stagnant one. It is a mind that is in the best possible condition to work, to think clearly and effectively.

Self-pity is a very common mental ill. Those who suffer much from this affliction usually have very good imagination. They think they are slighted and abused. They know that they do not get their dues. They envy others and are sure that others prosper at their expense. They minimize their blessings and magnify their misfortunes. This state of mind leads to spite and malice. These people become very nervous and irritable and are a nuisance, not only to themselves, but to those who are unfortunate enough to have to associate with them.

Self-consciousness and self-centeredness are twin evils. The sufferers lack perspective. They magnify their own importance. They believe they are the targets of many other minds and eyes. The youth refuses to take a dip in the ocean because he knows that the rest of the people on the beach are watching his spindle shanks or perhaps the bathing suit would reveal his narrow, undeveloped chest. The young man is afraid to go onto the dance floor because everybody is sure to see his ungainly gyrations. He stammers and stutters when he speaks because others are paying particular attention to his words, when in truth he is attracting little or no attention. Whether working or playing, those whose good opinions are worth having are too busy to spend much time in finding fault with others and discovering flaws that do not concern them. More enjoyment is to be had in looking at fine physiques and graceful movements than in watching the less favored.

We always do our best when we are natural. When we become self-conscious we become artificial and awkward. We can not even breathe properly. Those who are ever thinking about themselves fail to do things well enough to hold sustained attention, even if they are able to gain it for a while. Those who do their work well will in time gain the attention and appreciation they require. No one can long occupy a high place in the public heart without adding to the profit or pleasure of the world.

Here is a good line of thought for those who are too self-centered and self-important: "There are millions of solar systems in the universe, some of them much greater than ours. There are uncounted planets in space, beside some of which our little earth is a mere toy. Some of these planets are doubtless inhabited. Even on this small earth there are over a billion people. I am one in a number so great that my mind can not grasp such a multitude. Countless billions have gone before and they got along very well before I was born. Countless billions will live and die after I have passed on, and if they hear of me it will probably be by accident. And so it will be for ages and ages, so extensive that my brain can not grasp the stretch of time, which is without beginning and without end. How much do I, individually, amount to?"

And an honest answer must be, "Personally I am of very small importance."

An individual can not live of himself, for himself and by himself. Only as he adds his efforts to those of others does his work count. When we realize that we are but atoms in this vast universe, we get down to a business basis. Then it is easy to get adjusted. In order to count at all we must be in harmony with some of the rest of the atoms and when we discover this we are in a mental state to be of some real use. Building for individual glory is vanity. Sometimes an individual builds so well that he is picked out for special attention and honor, but this is comparatively seldom. As a rule, we can only help a little in shaping the ends of the race by adding our mite, as privates in the ranks. The time we spend in nursing our conceit is wasted.

This does not mean that we are worms in the dust. A human being is a paradox. He is so little, yet he has great possibilities. Our bodies are kept close to the earth, but our minds can be free and unfettered, soaring through time and space, exploring innumerable worlds of thought.

But it will not do to be too self-centered or consider one's self of too great importance, for this lessens one's chances of meriting the esteem of others.

The well balanced man is not greatly affected by too great praise or excessive censure, for he realizes that though the public may be hasty and unjust at times, in the end it renders a fairly just verdict.

Fear is one of the harmful negative or depressing emotions. Fear, like all other depressing emotions, poisons the body. This is not said in a figurative sense. It is an actual scientific fact; it has been demonstrated chemically. Were it not for the fact that the lungs, skin, kidneys and the bowels are constantly removing poisons from the body, an acute attack of fear would prove fatal.

Fear or fright is largely a habit. The parents are often responsible for this affliction. It is far too common for them to scare their children. They people the darkness with all kinds of danger and with horrible shapes, and the children, with their vivid imaginations, magnify these. Children should be taught to meet all conditions in life courageously and fear should not be instilled into their minds. There is a great deal of difference between fear and the caution which all must learn or perish early.

The caution that is implanted in the human breast is our heritage from the ages and works for our preservation. It was necessary during the infancy of the race when man had to struggle with the animals for supremacy. Beyond this point fear is a health-destroyer.

There are people who cultivate fear until they imagine they are ever in danger. They fear that they may lose their health, their mind, their good name. Some are afraid of many things. Others have one pet fear.

Today the fear of the unseen is strong in the public mind. I refer to the fear of germs, those tiny plants which are so small that the unaided eye can not see them. Children are shown moving pictures of these tiny beings, enormously enlarged and very formidable in appearance. They are told to beware, for these germs are in our food, in our drink, on the earth, in the air, in fact everywhere that man lives.

It is very harmful to scare the young thus, for it inhibits physical action and stunts the mind. How much better it would be to teach the children these truths about the germs: "Yes, there are germs in our foods and beverages. They are on the earth, in the water and in the air. They are necessary for our existence. If we take good care of our bodies and direct our minds in proper channels, these germs will not, in fact, can not harm us. If we do not take care of ourselves, but allow our bodies to fill with debris, the germs try to clean this away; they multiply and grow into great armies while doing it, for they thrive on waste. It is our fault, not the fault of the germs, that we allow our bodies to degenerate. The germs are our good friends and if we treat ourselves properly they will do all they can to help keep the water, the earth and the air in fit condition for our use."

Such teachings have the advantage of being true. They are helpful and healthful. The popular teachings are disease-producing. The mental depression and bodily inhibition caused by fear are injurious. Those who fear a certain kind of disease often bring this ill upon themselves, so powerful is suggestion. The fear is more dangerous than the thing feared.

In fear there is loss of both physical and mental power. Not only the voluntary muscles become impotent, but the involuntary ones lose in effectiveness. Digestion is partly or wholly suspended. "Scared stiff" is a popular and truthful expression. The bodily rhythm is lost, the breathing becomes jerky and the heart beats out of tune.

Keep fear out of the lives of babes. If children are taught the truth, there will be little fear in adult minds. Children should not be taught prayers in which there is an element of fear. It is much better to bring children up to love other people and God than to fear.

Those who have cultivated fear should try suggestion. Positive suggestion is always best. Let them analyze matters thus: "I have feared daily and nightly. Nothing has happened. I have brought much unnecessary discomfort upon myself. There is nothing to fear and I shall be brave hereafter." Those who fear God have a low conception of Him. Let them remember the beautiful saying that "God is love." Through repeating them often enough, such positive suggestions sink so deeply into the mind that they replace doubts and fears.

About 2500 years ago Pythagoras wrote: "Hate and fear breed a poison in the blood, which, if continued, affect eyes, ears, nose and the organs of digestion. Therefore, it is not wise to hear and remember the unkind things that others may say of us." Pythagoras was an ancient philosopher, but his words express modern scientific truths.

Worry: Worrying is perhaps the most common and the worst of our mental sins. Worry is like a cancer: It eats in and in. It is destructive of both body and mind. It is due largely to lack of self-control and is a symptom of cowardice. Much worry is also indicative of great selfishness, which most of those afflicted will deny. Those who worry much are always in poor health, which grows progressively worse. The form of indigestion accompanied by great acidity and gas formation is a prolific source of worry, as well as of other mental and physical troubles. The acidity irritates the nervous system and the irritation in time causes mental depression.

Confirmed worriers will worry about the weather, the past, the present, the future, about work and about play, about food, clothing and drink, about those who are present and those who are absent. Nothing escapes them and they bring sadness and woe in their wake.

Worrying is slow suicide.

Elbert Hubbard says that our most serious troubles are those that never happen.

Worrying is a very futile employment, for it never does any good, and it reacts evilly upon the one who indulges in it, and those with whom he associates. It is a waste of time and energy. The energy thus used could be directed into useful channels.

Let those who are afflicted with this bad and annoying habit get into good physical condition. Then many of the worries will take wing. If they persist, it would be well to face the matter frankly and honestly, setting down the advantages of worrying on one side and the disadvantages on the other. Then take into consideration that not one thing in a thousand worried about happens, and if something disagreeable does occur, worrying can not prevent it. Besides a disagreeable happening now and then will not cause half of the discomfort and trouble that a disturbed mind does.

"And this too shall pass away," is an ancient saying which it would be well to remember in conjunction with, "And this will probably never happen."

Anger is a form of temporary insanity. It is an emotion that is unbecoming in strong men, for it is a sign of weakness, and the women who indulge in it frequently can not long keep the respect of others. Those who become angry lay themselves open to wounds of all kinds, for they partly lose their mental and physical faculties temporarily. An angry man is easily vanquished in any contest where ready wit is necessary. As the saying is, he makes a fool of himself. To be high strung and quick to lose one's temper may sound fine in romantic rubbish, but in real life it is folly, for much more can be accomplished by being calm.

Like hatred, anger produces poisons in the system. An angry mother's milk has been known to kill the nursing child. A fit of anger is so serious that the evil effects can be felt for several days, and those who indulge in daily or even weekly loss of temper can not enjoy the best of health, for the anger produces enough toxins to poison all the fluids of the body.

Fortunately, anger is one of the emotions that can be conquered in a reasonable time, if there is a real desire to do so. It should not take an adult more than one or two years to get himself under control.

During anger there is a tensing of various muscles, those of the face and hands for instance. If this tensing is not allowed the anger will not last long. If there is a tendency to become angry, relax and the mind will ease up. A perfectly relaxed individual can not harbor anger, for this emotion requires tensing of body and mind. A determination to control the temper and a whole-hearted apology after each display of anger will prove very effective in reducing the frequency and force of the attacks. Mental suggestion is not as powerful as some say, but it is such a great force for good or evil, depending on its use, that those who are wise will not neglect it as a means of self-conquest.

People who are easily offended and "stand on their dignity," have a very poor footing. Those who find it necessary to inform others that they are ladies or gentlemen, are very apt to be prejudiced in their own favor. Gentlefolks do not need to advertise, nor do they do so. Others recognize their worth intuitively.

Fretting is anger on a small scale. It is a habit that is easily formed. The fretter and those about him are made uncomfortable. Those who respect themselves and others do not indulge.

Hatred is one of the most harmful and poisonous of emotions. Fortunately, violent hatred can last but a short time, otherwise it would prove fatal. Some are chronic haters. He who hates harms himself. The thoughts weave themselves into one's personality and form the character.

Jealousy is one of the most disagreeable of emotions. The jealous person insists on suffering. A jealous woman can convert a home into an inferno. Jealousy is sure to kill love in time. The jealous individual often excuses himself on the ground that he loves. That is not true. There is more fear than love at the base of jealousy. Jealous people are selfish and too indolent mentally to give their thoughts a positive direction.

Those who are violently jealous are suffering from mental aberration. The jealous person loses, for he drives away the object of his affection.

There are many jealous men, but women suffer most. Bad health and idleness are two prolific causes of jealousy. It has probably broken up more homes than any other one thing. It is blighting to all it touches.

Men and women may feel flattered for a time by producing jealousy, but it is a satisfaction of very short duration. They soon grow weary of the questions, doubts and reproaches.

Those who are sensible enough to give freely to others the liberty they crave for themselves do not suffer much from this emotion. It would help greatly if man and wife would look upon the marriage relation more as a partnership and less as a form of bondage. One of the partners can not force the other one to be "good." People do the best by others when full confidence is given, and even if the confidence should be misplaced, it would be better than to suffer from this corroding emotion at all times.

It is not an easy task to overcome jealousy, but it can be done within a reasonable time if there is a real desire. First get physical health. Then get busy with interesting, useful work. Get something worth while to occupy the mind and the hands. Determine to be master of yourself and not a slave to what is often but figments of the imagination. Unfortunately, jealousy so dwarfs the judgment at times that the sufferers seek only to rule or ruin. Love and hate are so closely akin that it is hard to find the dividing line.

Sorrow: Some dedicate their lives to a sorrow. They make martyrs of themselves. They have suffered a loss and they dwell upon it during all of their waking hours. It may be that it was a very ordinary or worthless husband or child. After death the poor real is converted into a glorious ideal. With the passing years the virtues of the departed grow. All the love and tenderness are lavished upon the dead and the living are neglected. It is generally women who suffer from this peculiar form of mild insanity, but men are not exempt.

It is natural to feel the loss of a dear one, but so long as we are mortal we must accept these things as matters of course.

Related to this form of sorrow is the regretting or brooding over past actions, especially in connection with the dead. Perhaps something that should have been done was neglected, or something was done that should have been left undone. Over this the sufferer broods by the hour, leading to a form of sad resignation that is rather irritating to normal people.

For such people a change of interest and a change of scene will often prove very beneficial.

Envy and spite are closely akin to jealousy and anger. They have the same effect in lesser degree.

Vacillation of mind is a common fault. Many small questions have to be settled and a few important ones. Some are in the habit of deferring their decisions from time to time, or making and revoking their decisions. Then they decide over again, after which there is another revocation. This is repeated until it is absolutely necessary to make a final decision. By this time the mind is so muddled that the chances are that the last decision will be inferior to the first one. No one who leads an active life can be right all the time. He who is right six times out of ten does pretty well, and he who can make a correct decision three times out of four can command a fine salary as an executive or build up a flourishing business of his own, if his mind is active.

The doubt and uncertainty which result from unsettled questions, which should be promptly decided, are more harmful than an occasional error. The untroubled mind works most quickly and truly.

Related to this in minor key is the doubtful condition of mind where the individual has to do things several times before he is sure they are properly done. For instance, there is the man who must try the office door several times to be sure that it is locked and after being satisfied on this point he is obliged to unlock it and investigate the condition of the safe door. Then it is necessary to attend to the office door two or three times again. This kind of doubtfulness takes many forms. It does no special harm except that it leads to much waste of time. Such people should teach themselves concentration, thinking about one thing only at a time, until they learn that when a thing is done it is properly done.

Judging: Many insist on passing judgment on everything and everybody that come to their notice. Every individual has to be placed with the sheep or the goats. This is a great waste of time. Each one of us can know so little about the majority of individuals we meet and of the vast volume of knowledge that is to be had that if we try to judge everyone and everything, our opinions become worthless. Wise people are never afraid to say, "I don't know." If it is necessary to judge, let there be kindness.

Volunteering advice: This is another annoying habit. It is very well to give advice if it is desired and asked for, otherwise it is a waste of time. Take a person with a cold, for example: If he meets twenty people he may be told of fifteen different cures for it, ranging from goose grease on a red rag to suggestive therapeutics. If he were to act upon all the advice received there would probably be a funeral. It is best to be sparing with advice. Those who have any that is worth while will be asked for it and paid for their trouble. Free advice is generally worth what it costs.

Cranks: Many allow themselves to get into a mental rut with their thoughts running almost entirely to one subject. This is a mild form of insanity, for normal people have many interests. These people are the cranks. They can talk volumes about their favorite topic, often of no importance. It may be some peculiar religion or ethics; or that Bacon wrote the plays of Shakespeare; or some health fad, or almost any subject.

Of all the cranks the diet crank is one of the most annoying, for he has three good opportunities to air his views each day. With the best meaning in the world he does more harm to the cause of food reform than do the advocates of living in the good old way, eating, drinking and being merry and dying young. When people become possessed of too much zeal and enthusiasm regarding a subject, they are sure that their knowledge is the truth and they insist upon trying to enforce their way upon others, resent having their old habits interfered with forcibly. Those who are too persistent and insistent produce antagonism and prejudice in the minds of others, and then it is almost impossible to impart the truth to them, for they will neither see nor hear.

To be able to influence others for better is a grand and glorious thing, but it is well to remember that we can not force knowledge which is contrary to popular thought upon others suddenly. Those who change a well rooted opinion generally do so gradually. When they first hear the truth, they say it is ridiculous. After a while they think there may be something in it. At last they see its superiority over their former opinions and accept it. It requires infinite patience on the part of the educators to impart unpopular knowledge to other adults, no matter how much truth it contains.

The truth about physical well-being is so simple and so self-evident that it is exceptionally hard to get an unprejudiced audience. From the time when the ancient heathen priests were the healers until today the impression has been that health and healing are beyond the understanding of the common mind, and therefore people are willing to be mystified. The mysterious has such a strong appeal in this world of uncertainties that it is more attractive than the simple truth. Mystery simply demands faith. The truth compels thinking and thoughts are often painful.

By all means, avoid being overinsistent in trying to impart health knowledge to others. All who have a little knowledge of the fundamentals of health and growth know that useful men and women are going into degeneration and premature death constantly, because of violated health laws. If these people on the brink, who can yet be saved by natural means, are told how it can be done, they generally either refuse to believe it, or they have led such self-indulgent lives that it is beyond their power to change. The knowledge often comes too late.

Those who are anxious to do good in the spreading of health knowledge among their friends can serve best by getting health themselves. If a physical wreck evolves into good health there will be considerable comment and inquiry. This is the opportunity to tell what nature will do and inform others where to obtain a good interpretation of nature's workings.

A little practicing is worth more than a great deal of preaching. The truth is the truth, no matter what the source, but it is more effective if it comes from one who lives it.

I have gone into the subject of health cranks so deeply because there are so many of them. They get a little knowledge and then they believe they are masters of the subject. The right attitude toward proper living, and especially toward proper eating is: "I shall try to conduct myself so as to be healthy and efficient. If others desire my help, I shall try to indicate the way to them. Right living is no sign of superior goodness or merit, being a matter of higher selfishness, so I deserve no credit for it. Although health is very important, I shall refrain from attempting to force my will on others."

After conquering ourselves it is time to begin making foreign conquests, but by that time the realization comes that in the end it is best to leave others free to work out their own salvation. The desire is strong to mould others according to our pattern, but those who size themselves up honestly soon come to the conclusion that they are so imperfect that perchance some other pattern is fully as good.

Postponing happiness: One peculiar state of mind is to refuse to be happy at present. The romantic girl and boy think they can not be happy until they are married. After marriage they find that they have to gain a certain amount of wealth before happiness comes. Then they have to postpone it for social position. They continue postponing happiness from time to time and the result is that they never attain it. Happiness is not a great entity that bursts upon us, transforming us into radiant beings. It is a comfortable feeling that brings peace and places us in harmony with our surroundings. It can best be gained by doing well each day the work that is to be done, cheerfully giving in return for what is received. Happiness is largely a habit. It is as easy to be bright and cheerful as it is to be sad and doleful, and much more comfortable. If we look for the best we will find beauty even in the most unpromising places. If we are looking for tears and woe, we can easily find them.

We can get along without happiness, but it adds so much color and beauty to life, it makes us so much better, it helps us so much to be useful that it is folly to do without it. It is not gained by narrow selfishness. Those who forget themselves most and are kind and considerate find it. By giving it to others we get it for ourselves. Ecstasy and rapture are emotions of short duration. They are so exhilarating that they soon wear out.

We all have our little troubles and annoyances. These we should accept as inevitable, and neither think nor talk much about them. They help to wear away the rough edges. We are stupid at times and so are others and then mistakes are made. These should also be accepted as inevitable, and we should not be more annoyed by those that others make than by our own. Those who go into a rage when their subordinates err waste much time and energy, erring gravely themselves.

It is not necessary to notice every unimportant detail that is not pleasing. Fault-finding, carping and nagging destroy harmony. Disagreements about trifles often lead to broken friendship and enmity. Most quarrels are about trifles.

If mistakes are made, learn the lesson they teach and then forget about them. All live, active beings make mistakes. Sometimes we make serious ones and afterwards regrets come, but these must soon be thrust aside. Brooding has put many into the insane asylums.

Introspection: It is not well to allow the mind to dwell upon one's self very much. Give yourself enough thought to guide yourself through life, and then for the rest apply the mind to work and play. Many of those who are too self-centered end up in believing they are something or somebody else and then they are shut away from the public.

Introspection is a very useless employment. Individually we are so small, and the mind has such great possibilities, that if we center it upon our tiny physical being, things become unbalanced and the mind ceases to work to good advantage. It is useless to go deeply into self-analysis, for we are very poor judges of ourselves. One of my neighbors delved so deeply into his heart and tried so hard to find out if he was fit to dwell in heaven that he lost his mind and had to be confined for a long time. He allowed his vision to narrow down to one subject. There are many subjects that lead to insanity if they are allowed exclusive possession of the mind.

After we have given ourselves proper care, we should think no more about ourselves. The best way is to get busy in work and play and forget ourselves. It is much better to love others than to center our love upon ourselves. If we conduct ourselves well we shall have all the love from others that we need. If there is a tendency to be introspective, cure it by becoming active mentally and physically.

Those who have acquired the bad habit of thinking and talking ill of others should break themselves of it. First cease talking ill. Then begin to look for the good points and mention them. By and by the thoughts will be good. Those who lack a virtue can often cultivate it by assuming it.

One of the most helpful things is a sense of humor. Laughter brings about relaxation and relaxation gives ease of body and mind. He who can see his own weaknesses and smile at them is surely safe and sane. If the mind is too austere, cultivate a sense of humor. Train yourself to appreciate the ridiculous appearance you make and instead of being chagrined, smile. When others laugh at you, join them.

Whatever the mental ill may be, one-half of its cure will be brought about by getting physical health.

Be charitable, tolerant and kind, and the good things in life will come to you. Be slow to judge and slower still to condemn others.

Those who give love attract it. Hypatia said: "Express beauty in your lives and beauty flows to you and through you. To love means to be loved, and to put hate behind is the sum of all loving that is of any avail."

The best "New Thought" is the best old thought. If we only would put some of the beautiful knowledge into common use, what an agreeable dwelling place this world would be. Marcus Aurelius gave us this pearl of wisdom: "When you arise in the morning, think what a precious privilege it is to live, to breathe, to think, to enjoy, to love! God's spirit is close to us when we love. Therefore it is better not to resent, not to hate, not to fear. Equanimity and moderation are the secrets of power and peace."

CHAPTER III.

FOOD.

The human body is so wonderfully made that as yet we have only a poor understanding of it, but we are learning a little each decade, and perhaps in time we shall have a fair knowledge both of the body and of the mind. Body and mind can not be considered as two separate entities, for neither one is of any use without the other.

The body is not a machine. Those who look upon it as such make the mistake of feeding it as they would an engine, thinking that it takes so much fuel to keep going. The human organism is perhaps never quite alike on any two consecutive days, for the body changes with our thoughts, actions and environment, and the conditions never quite repeat themselves and therefore we have to readjust ourselves.

The most important single item for gaining and retaining physical health is proper feeding, yet the medical men of this country pay so little attention to this subject that in some of our best equipped medical colleges dietetics are not taught. A total of from sixteen to thirty hours is considered sufficient to fit the future physicians to guide their patients in the selection, combination and preparation of food. Dietetics should be the principal subject of study. It should be approached both from the scientific and from the empirical side. It is not a rigid subject, but one which can be treated in a very elastic way. The scientific part is important, but the practical part, which is the art, is vastly more important. A part of the art of feeding and fasting is scientific, for we get the same results every time, under given conditions.

When we consider the fact that the body is made up of various tissues, such as connective tissue, blood, nerves and muscles; that these in turn are made up of billions of cells, as are the various glandular organs and membranes; that these cells are constantly bathed in blood and lymph, from which they select the food they need and throw the refuse away, we must marvel that an organism so complex is so resistant, stable and strong.

All articles of good quality are made by first-class workmen from fine materials. However, many people fail to realize that in order to have quality bodies they must take quality food, properly cooked or prepared, in the right proportions and combinations. If we feed the body properly, nature is kind enough to do good constructive work without any thought on our part.

You will find no rigid rules in these talks on diet, but you will find information that will enable you to select foods that will agree with you. People may well disagree on what to eat, for there are so many foods that a person could do without nine-tenths of them and still be well nourished. In fact, we consume too great a variety of food for our physical well-being. Great variety leads to overeating.

A healthy human body is composed of the following compounds, in about the proportions given:

Water, 60 to 65 per cent. Mineral matter, 5 to 6 per cent. Protein, 18 to 20 per cent. Carbohydrates, 1 per cent. Fat, 10 per cent. This is perhaps excessive.

These substances are very complex and well distributed throughout the body. They are composed of about sixteen or seventeen elements, but a pure element is very rarely found in the body, unless it be a foreign substance, such as mercury or lead. About 70 per cent of the body is oxygen, which is also the most abundant element of the earth. Then in order of their weight come carbon, hydrogen, nitrogen, calcium, phosphorus, sulphur, sodium, chlorine, fluorine, potassium, iron, magnesium and silicon.

Because it will be helpful in giving a better idea of the necessity for proper feeding, I shall devote a few words to each of these elements.

Oxygen is a colorless, tasteless, odorless gas, forming a large part of the atmospheric air, of water, of the earth's crust and of our foods. It is absolutely essential to life, for without oxygen there can be no combustion in the animal tissues, and without combustion there can be no life. The union of oxygen with fats, carbohydrates and proteins in the body results in slow combustion, which produces heat and energy. Our chief supply of oxygen comes directly from the air, but this is supplemented by the intake in food and water.

Carbon is the chief producer of energy within the body, being the principal constituent of starches, sugars and fats. It is what we rely on for internal heat, as well as for heating our dwellings, for the essential part of coal is carbon. The carbonaceous substances are needed in greater quantity than any other, but if they are taken pure, they cause starvation more quickly than if no food were eaten. This has been proved through experiments in feeding nothing but refined sugar, which is practically pure carbon. Salts and nitrogenous foods are essential to life.

Hydrogen is a very light gas, without odor, taste or color. It is a necessary constituent of all growing, living things. It is plentifully supplied in water. All acids contain hydrogen and so does the protoplasm of the body.

Nitrogen is also a colorless, tasteless, odorless gas. It is an essential constituent of the body, being present in all compounds of protein. It is abundant in the atmospheric air, from which it is taken by plants. We get our supply either directly from vegetable foods or from animal products, such as milk, eggs and meat.

Calcium is needed principally for the bones and for the teeth, but it is also necessary in the blood, where it assists in coagulation. We get sufficient calcium salts in fruits, grains and vegetables, provided they are properly prepared. The conventional preparation of the food often results in the loss of the various salts, which causes tissue degeneration. If the supply of calcium in the food is too small, the bones and the teeth suffer, for the blood removes the calcium from these structures. Growing children need more calcium proportionately than do adults. This is without doubt the reason pregnant women suffer so much from softening of the teeth. They are fed on foods robbed of their calcium, such as white bread and vegetables that have been drained.

Phosphorus in some forms is a poison whether taken in solid compounds or inhaled in fumes, producing phossy jaw. In other forms it is indispensable for bodily development. The compounds of phosphorus are present in fats, bones and protein. In natural foods they are abundantly present, but when these foods are unduly refined, or are soaked in water which is thrown away, much of the phosphorus is lost. We get phosphorus from milk, eggs, cereals, legumes and other foods. Of course, there is phosphorus in fish, but those who eat sea food to make themselves brainy will probably be disappointed. Phosphates are necessary for brain development, but those who eat natural foods never need to go to the trouble of taking special foods for the brain. If the rest of the body is well nourished, the brain will have sufficient food, and if the body is poorly nourished the brain will suffer.

Sulphur is present in protein and we get a sufficient supply from milk, meat and legumes. The element sulphur is quite inert and harmless, but some of its acids and salts are very poisonous. Sulphur dioxide is freely used in the process of drying fruits, as a bleacher. In this form it is poisonous, and for that reason it would be well to avoid bleached dried fruits. We need some sulphur, but not in the form of sulphur dioxide or concentrated sulphurous acid, both of which are used in the manufacture of food.

Sodium, in its elementary state, which is not found in nature, is a white, silvery metal. It is found in great abundance in the succulent vegetables, and is present in practically all foods. As sodium chloride, or common table salt, it is taken in great quantities by most people. Those who have no salt get along well without it, which shows that it is not needed in large amounts. If but a little is added to the food, it does no perceptible harm, but when sprinkled on everything that is eaten, from watermelons to meat, it is without doubt harmful. By soaking foods, they are deprived of much of their soda: The two sodium salts that are very abundant are sodium chloride, or common salt, and sodium carbonate, generally called soda.

Chlorine is ordinarily combined in our foods with sodium or potash, forming the chlorides. It is essential to life. He who gets enough sodium also gets enough chlorine. In its elementary form it is an irritating gas, used for bleaching purposes.

Fluorine is present in small quantities in the body, appearing as fluorides in the bones and teeth. It is supplied by the various foods. In its elementary form it is a poisonous gas.

Potassium is found in the body in very small quantities, but it is very important. It is mostly in the form of potassium phosphate in the muscles and in the blood. It is necessary for muscular activity. It is found in most foods in greater abundance than is sodium, which indicates that it plays an important part in development. Like sodium, it is easily dissolved out of foods which are soaked in water, and this is one of the reasons that vegetables should not be soaked and the water thrown away. It is very peculiar in its metallic state, being a silvery metal, very light in weight, which burns when thrown upon water. That is, it decomposes both itself and the water with the liberation of so much heat that it fires the escaping hydrogen, which burns with a violet flame. Pure potassium is not found in nature.

Iron is found in very small quantities in the human body, but it is absolutely essential to life. Animals deprived of iron die in a few weeks, and people will do the same under similar circumstances. Iron is obtained principally from fruits and vegetables, but it is also present in other foods. Man can not make use of inorganic iron. He has to get his supply from the vegetable and animal kingdoms. The giving of inorganic iron is folly and helps to ruin the teeth and the stomach of the one who takes it. In the form of hemoglobin this element is the chief agent in carrying oxygen from the lungs to the tissues of the body. In the manufacture of foods, much of the iron is lost. For instance, whole wheat flour contains about ten times as much iron as does the white flour. Too little iron causes, among other ills, anemia, and if the iron is very low, chlorosis or the green sickness may ensue.

Magnesium is found principally as phosphate in the bones. It is present both in animal and vegetable foods. Its function in the body is not well understood, but it appears to assist the phosphorus.

Silicon is found in traces in the human body. It is supplied in small quantities in nearly all of our foods, and therefore we must take it for granted that it is necessary, although we are in the dark as to its uses. It is very abundant in various rocks. The cereals are especially rich in silicon. In wheat it is found in the bran and is removed from the white flour.

The elements mentioned are the most important in the body, though others are found in traces. We do not find the elements present as elements, but in the form of very complex compounds. Under our present conditions of living, we generally partake of too much carbonaceous and nitrogenous food, and get too little of the salts, except sodium chloride, which is taken in too great quantity. Salt, to most people, means but one thing, sodium chloride or table salt. However, there are thousands of salts, and when salts are mentioned in this book, all those necessary for the processes of life are meant, whether they be compounds of fluorine, sulphur, phosphorus, calcium, iron or magnesium or other metals and minerals.

Salts are not usually classified as foods, but they are essential to life. Supply the body with all the protein, sugar, starch and fat that it requires, but withhold the salts, and it is but a question of a few weeks before life ceases.

This is why it is so important to improve our methods of cooking. A potato that is peeled, soaked in cold water and boiled, may lose as much as one-half of its salts, according to one of the bulletins sent out by the U. S. Department of Agriculture. Other vegetables not only lose their salts by such treatment, but as high as 30 per cent of their nutritive value.

The lesson we should learn from this is that ordinarily if it is necessary to soak foods, such as beans, they should be cooked in the water in which they have been soaked. Furthermore, where possible, as it is with nearly all succulent vegetables, we should take the fluid in which the vegetables have been cooked as a part of the meal. If the vegetables are properly cooked, there will not be much fluid to take. To pour away the water in which vegetables have been cooked means that perhaps one-third of the food value and one-third to one-half of the valuable salts are lost. Why continue impoverishing foods in this way?

Dr. Charles Page deserves much credit for calling our attention to this fact when most healers neither thought nor talked about it. Now all up-to-date healers with a knowledge of dietetics realize how important it is to give good food. For those who wish more detailed information on the composition of the salts, I insert a table which was compiled by Otto Carque and published in "Brain and Brawn," February, 1913. Those who wish still more detailed knowledge can find it in volumes on food analysis and in some government reports.

MINERAL MATTER IN 1000 PARTS OF WATER-FREE FOOD PRODUCTS.
==
=========== P P M h o a o C t C g s S S h a S a n p u i l s o l e h l l o s d c s l o p
i r i i i i r r h c i u u u u o u u o n m m m m n s r n e Total| | | | | | | | | Salts|
K2O |Na2O | CaO | MgO |Fe2O3|P2O5 | SO2 |SiO2 | Cl --------------------------
-- Human milk 34.70|11.73| 3.16| 5.80|
0.75| 0.07| 7.84| 0.33| 0.07| 6.38 Cow's milk 55.30|13.70| 5.34|12.24|
1.69| 0.30|15.79| 0.17| 0.02| 8.04 Meat (avge) 40.00|16.52| 1.44| 1.12|
1.28| 0.28|17.00| 0.64| 0.44| 1.56 Eggs 41.80| 6.27| 9.56| 4.56| 0.46|
0.17|15.72| 0.13| 0.13| 3.72 Seafish 84.20|18.35|12.55|12.80| 3.28|
....|32.13| ....| ....| 9.60 Cottage Cheese 64.30| 8.50| 0.90|22.50| 1.50|
0.50|24.35| 0.10| ....|11.20 | | | | | | | | | Apples 33.00|11.78|8.61| 1.35|
2.89| 0.46| 4.52| 2.01| 1.42| .... Strawberries 65.00|13.72|18.53| 9.23| ....|

3.73| 7.97| 2.05| 7.82| 1.10 Gooseberries 29.00|11.22| 2.87| 3.54| 1.70|
1.32| 5.71| 1.71| 0.75| 0.22 Prunes 37.75|18.28| 3.41| 4.34| 1.36| 0.94|
6.03| 1.21| 1.19| 0.15 Peaches 17.60| 9.63| 1.50| 1.41| 0.92| 0.18| 2.67|
1.00| 0.26| .... Cherries 34.60|17.94| 0.76| 2.60| 1.90| 0.69| 5.54| 1.76|
3.11| 0.46 Grapes 25.20|14.16| 0.35| 2.72| 1.06| 0.45| 3.93| 1.41| 0.70|
0.38 Figs 41.00|11.63|10.77| 7.75| 3.78| 0.60| 0.53| 2.77| 2.43| 1.10 Olives
33.40|27.02| 2.52| 2.49| 0.06| 0.31| 0.46| 0.36| 0.22| 0.06 Apricots
33.60|19.68| 3.76| 1.08| 2.89| 0.46| 4.52| 2.01| 1.42| .... Pears
25.60|14.00| 2.17| 2.05| 1.52| 0.25| 3.90| 1.45| 0.38| .... Watermelons
40.00|18.00| 3.75| 4.00| 2.10| 1.75| 5.60| 2.10| 7.60| 1.10 Bananas
32.40|16.20| 0.80| 0.25| 0.32| 0.10| 2.03| 0.21| ....| 2.47 Oranges
38.15|18.62| 0.95| 8.65| 2.03| 0.38| 4.70| 2.00| 0.25| 0.29 | | | | | | | | |
Spinach 191.00|21.71|57.42|22.73|12.22| 6.40|19.58|13.18| 8.60|12.03
Onions 48.40|12.10| 1.55|10.65| 2.55| 2.20| 7.25| 2.65| 8.10| 1.35 Carrots
69.00|25.46|14.63| 7.80| 3.04| 0.70| 8.83| 4.45| 1.66| 3.18 Asparagus
86.40|20.74|14.77| 9.33| 3.72| 2.94|16.07| 5.36| 9.50| 5.10 Radishes
110.40|35.33|23.37|15.45| 3.42| 3.09|12.03| 7.18| 1.00|10.10 Cauliflower
91.20|40.46| 5.38| 5.10| 3.37| 0.91|18.42|11.86| 3.37| 3.10 Cucumbers
100.00|41.20|10.00| 7.30| 4.15| 1.40|20.20| 6.90| 8.00| 6.60 Lettuce
180.70|67.94|13.55|26.56|11.20| 9.40|16.62| 6.87|14.64|13.82 Potatoes
44.20|26.56| 1.33| 1.15| 2.18| 0.48| 7.47| 2.89| 0.88| 1.55 Cabbage
123.00|45.33|11.68|21.65| 4.90| 0.86|11.07|17.10| 1.10|10.45 Tomatoes
176.00|82.50|32.90|11.35|13.55| 1.00|10.75| 5.00| 7.75|18.00 Red Beets
41.65| 8.45|21.60| 2.50| 0.10| 1.00| 2.55| 0.50| 2.00| 2.95 Celery
180.00|48.60|65.25|14.70| 6.75| 1.60|14.50| 6.50| 4.30|17.80 | | | | | | |
| | Walnuts 17.40| 2.20| 0.17| 0.97| 2.88| 0.61|10.10| 0.22| 0.12| 0.12
Almonds 21.00| 2.31| 0.38| 3.04| 3.95| 0.23|10.10| 0.96| 0.04| 0.06
Cocoanuts 18.70| 8.21| 1.57| 8.60| 1.76| ....| 2.18| 0.95| 0.09| 2.50 | | | | |
| | | | Lentils 34.70|12.08| 4.62| 2.18| 0.87| 0.69|12.60| ....| ....| 1.61 Peas
30.03|13.06| 0.30| 1.45| 2.42| 0.24|10.87| 1.03| 0.27| 0.53 Beans
38.20|15.85| 0.42| 1.91| 2.73| 0.19|14.86| 1.30| 0.25| 0.69 Peanuts 24.30|
9.27| 0.21| 0.95| 2.29| 0.27|10.60| 0.45| 0.05| 0.23 | | | | | | | | | | Whole
Wheat 23.10| 7.20| 0.50| 0.75| 2.80| 0.30|10.90| 0.09| 0.46| 0.07 White
flour 5.70| 1.82| 0.08| 0.43| 0.44| 0.03| 2.80| ....| ....| .... Rye 21.30| 6.84|
0.31| 0.61| 2.39| 0.25|10.16| 0.28| 0.30| 0.01 Barley 31.30| 5.10| 1.28|
0.02| 3.92| 0.53|10.27| 0.93| 8.98| .... Oats 34.50| 6.18| 0.59| 1.24| 2.45|
0.41| 8.83| 0.62|13.52| 0.03 Corn 18.50| 5.50| 0.02| 0.04| 2.87| 0.15|
8.44| 0.15| 0.39| 0.35 Whole Rice 16.00| 3.60| 0.67| 0.59| 1.78| 0.22|

8.60| 0.08| 0.42| 0.02 Rice, polished 4.00| 0.87| 0.22| 0.13| 0.45| 0.05| 2.15| 0.03| 0.11| 0.01 --

Please remember that most of the salts must be worked into organic form for us by vegetation, and that we are able to take but few elements that have not been thus elaborated.

We need a moderate amount of food to maintain the body in health, but we should be careful not to overindulge.

Perhaps the most injurious errors are made by people who eat because they wish to gain in weight. They consider themselves below weight and they try to force a gain by overeating. This is a serious mistake and leads to much suffering.

There is no weight that can be called ideal for all people. To get a basis, I copy a table from the literature of an insurance company. This is for people twenty years old:

Height Weight 5--0........114 1........117 2........121 3........124 4........128 5........132 6........136 7........140 8........144 9........149 10........153 11........158 6--0........162 1........167 2........172 3........177

If the weight is much above this, it is a sure sign that the individual is building disease. It may be Bright's disease, fatty heart, arteriosclerosis, cancer or any other ill. The muscles can not be increased in size very much by eating and there is a limit to the amount of fluid that can be stored away. Stout people generally carry about a great amount of fat.

Excess of fat is a burden. It replaces other tissues and weakens the muscles. It overcrowds the abdominal and thoracic cavities, thus making the breath short and the working of the heart more difficult, also producing a tendency to prolapsus of the various abdominal organs.

People make the mistake of thinking that stoutness indicates health. It indicates disease. Going into weight is going into degeneration. Women like to be plump for various reasons, some of which are not the most creditable to either men or women. Fat people are not good looking. There is not a statue in the world sculptured on corpulent lines that is considered beautiful.

It is natural for some people to be slender and for others to be rather plump, but fatness is abnormal. Rolling double chins and protruding abdomens are signs of self-abuse in eating and drinking. As a rule women are at their right weight at twenty and men at twenty-two or twenty-three. This weight they should retain. If twenty or thirty pounds are added to it life will be materially shortened.

Perfect health is impossible for obese people, but it is within the reach of lean ones. In getting well, it is often necessary to become quite slender, but after the system has cleansed itself, it gains in weight again. It may take from several months to several years to obtain a normal weight after the ravages of disease. A healthy body is self-regulating and will be as heavy as it ought to be.

Those who eat too much in order to gain weight sometimes wreck their digestive and assimilative powers to such an extent that they lose a great deal of weight, and the more they eat the more they lose. Then it is necessary to reduce the food intake until digestion and assimilation catch up with supply. Then if the eating is right the individual goes to the proper weight and retains it.

The slender people are in the safest physical condition. The vast amount of statistics gathered by the life insurance companies bears this out. Remember that fat is a low grade tissue, which sometimes crowds out high grade tissue, that an excess indicates degeneration and that obesity is a disease. All fat people eat too much, even though they consider themselves small eaters. They should regulate their eating and drinking so that they will return to a normal weight. This is the only safe way to reduce.

Pay no attention to underweight. Eat what the body requires and is able to digest and assimilate, without causing any inconvenience. The organism will take care of the rest. To attempt to force weight onto a body at the expense of discomfort, disease, reduced efficiency and premature death shows poor judgment.

Losing weight does not matter at all if there is no discomfort or disease. It is all right to be a little lighter during summer than in winter.

In discussing food and its use, two words are frequently employed, digestion and fermentation. Strictly speaking, digestion is largely a process of fermentation, consisting of the breaking down of complex substances into simple ones, by means of ferments. However, in the popular mind digestion and fermentation are not synonymous, and will not be so considered in this book. To make my meaning clear, in this book the words will have the following meaning:

Digestion--the normal breaking down of food and formation into substances that can be used by the blood for building, repairing and producing heat and energy.

Fermentation--the abnormal breaking down of food in the digestive tract, producing discomfort and health impaired. This process manifests in various ways, such as the production of much gas in the digestive tract or hyperacidity of the body.

We will consider digestion as a process conducive to health, but fermentation, as one that leads to disease, being an early stage of digestive derangement.

CHAPTER IV.

OVEREATING.

All agree that excessive indulgence in alcoholics is harmful physically, mentally and morally. We condemn the too free use of tea and coffee and nearly all other excesses. However, intemperate eating is considered respectable. A large part of our social life consists in partaking of too much food.

Medical text-books say that we must eat great quantities of food to maintain strength and health. Humanity views the subject of eating from the wrong angle, and it will perhaps be many years before the majority gets the right point of view. We should eat to live, but most of us eat to die. Benjamin Franklin said that we dig our graves with our teeth.

Men and women band themselves into societies and associations for the purpose of decreasing or doing away with the use of tobacco and alcoholic drinks. They advocate temperance and even abstinence in the use of those things which do not appeal to their own senses; but most of them are far from temperate in their eating. They have very keen vision when searching for weaknesses and faults in others, but are quite near-sighted regarding their own.

Is excessive indulgence in liquor any worse than overeating? Not according to nature's answer. The inebriate deteriorates and so does the glutton. Both cause race deterioration. Gluttony is more common than inebriety and is responsible for more ills. Gluttony is often the cause of the tea, coffee, alcohol and drug habits. Overeating often causes so much irritation that food does not satisfy the cravings, and then drugs are used.

Improper eating, chiefly overeating, causes most of the ills to which man is heir. If people would learn to be moderate in all things disease and early death would be very rare.

It is quite important to combine foods properly, but the worst combinations of food eaten in moderation are harmless, as compared to the damage done by overeating of the best foods. Overeating is with us from the cradle to the grave. It shortens our days and fills them with woe.

There is a hoary belief that a pregnant woman must eat for two. The mothers have generally obeyed this dictum. The result is that women suffer greatly during pregnancy and at childbirth. The morning sickness, the aching back, the headache, the swollen legs and all of the discomforts and diseases from which civilized woman suffers during this period are mostly due to improper eating. Pregnancy and childbirth are physiologic and are devoid of any great amount of discomfort, pain or danger when women lead normal lives.

The overeating affects both mother and child. The mothers are often injured or lose their lives during childbirth. Sometimes labor is so protracted that the child dies and at other times the baby is so large that it can not be born naturally. The mother's suffering is frequently very great. In fact, it is at times so great that it is like a threatening storm cloud to many women, and some of them refuse to become mothers for this reason.

Babies born of normal mothers, who have lived moderately on a non-stimulating diet during gestation, are small. They rarely weigh more than six pounds. Their bones are flexible. The skull can easily be moulded because the bones are very cartilaginous. The result is that childbirth is rapid and practically devoid of pain. However, there are very few normal mothers, and consequently normal babies are also rare.

A heavy baby is never healthy. Its growth has been forced by excessive maternal feeding. It is no hardier than other growing things which result from hot-house methods. Such babies show early signs of catarrhal afflictions, indigestion or skin disease. Their bodies are filled with poisons before they are born.

Mothers who overeat invariably overfeed their babies. And why should they do otherwise? Family, friends and physicians give the same advice: The mother must eat much to be able to feed the child, and the child must be fed frequently in order to grow. It sounds very plausible, but it does not work well in practice.

Why are babies cross? Why do they soon show catarrhal symptoms? Why do they vomit so much? Why are they so subject to stomach and intestinal disorders? Why do they have skin eruptions? Because they are overfed.

The diseases of babies are almost entirely of digestive origin, and in nearly every instance overfeeding is the cause. Statistics show that about one-fifth of the babies born die before they are one year old. In nearly every instance the parents are to blame. One's intentions may be good, but good intentions coupled with wrong actions are deadly to infants. Oscar Wilde wrote, "We kill the thing we love." Parental love too often takes the form of indulging them and so it happens that hundreds of thousands of little ones are placed in their coffins annually through love.

Each year about 280,000 babies under one year of age perish in the United States, according to estimates based on census figures. Outside of accidental deaths, which are but a small per cent., the mortality should be practically nil. It is natural for children to be well, and healthy children do not die. If an army of about 280,000 of our men and women were to perish in a spectacular manner each year it would cause such sorrow and indignation that a remedy would soon be found. But we are so accustomed to the procession of little caskets to the grave that it hardly arouses comment. It costs too much in every way to produce life to waste it so lavishly.

Why do little children suffer so much from eruptive diseases, whooping cough, tonsilitis, adenoids, diphtheria and numerous other diseases? Because they are overfed. The younger the child the greater is the per cent. of disease due to wrong feeding. In adult life overeating and eating improperly otherwise are still the principal causes of disease. But during adult life the causation of disease is more complex than in childhood, for the senses have been more fully developed and instead of confining our physical sins to overeating we fall prey to the abuse of various appetites and passions.

Vigorous adults are often the victims of pneumonia, typhoid fever and tuberculosis. Overeating is chiefly to blame, not the bacteria which are given as the principal cause.

Rheumatism, kidney disease and diseases that manifest in hardening of the various tissues, all being forms of degeneration, are quite common. Again, the principal cause is overeating.

There are a great number of people who live many years without any special disease, but who are always on the brink of being ill. They are full-blooded and too corpulent. Although they are often considered successful, they are never fully efficient either physically or mentally. They do not know what good health is, but they are so accustomed to their state of toleration that they consider themselves healthy. They are rather proud of their stoutness and their friends mistake their precarious condition for health. These people often die suddenly, and friends and acquaintances are very much surprised. No healthy man dies suddenly and unexpectedly except by accident.

Instead of growing old gracefully, in possession of our senses and faculties, we die prematurely or go into physical and mental decay. Bleary eyes, pettiness, childishness and lost mental faculties are no part of nature's plan for advanced years. Those manifestations result from man's improvement on nature!

From birth to death we are victims of this terrible ogre of overeating. It deprives us of friends and relatives. It takes away our strength and health. It makes us mentally inefficient and cowardly. At last it deprives us of life when our work is not half done and our days should not be half run.

How is it possible, you may ask, that this is true? Of course, overeating is not the only cause, but it is the overwhelming one. It is the basic cause. Aided by other bad habits it conquers us. We are what we are because of our parentage, plus what we eat, drink, breathe and think, and the eating largely influences the other factors of life.

Cholera infantum causes the death of many babies. It never occurs in babies who are fed moderately on natural, clean food, not to exceed three or four times a day. The child is cross. The mother thinks that it is cross because it is hungry and accordingly feeds. The real cause of the irritability is the overfeeding that has already taken place. The baby has had so much milk that it is unable to digest all of it. A part of the milk spoils in the digestive tract. This fermented material is partly absorbed and irritates the whole system. A part of it remains in the alimentary tract where it acts as a direct local irritant to the intestines. When these are irritated, the blood-vessels begin to pour out their serum to soothe the bowels and the result is diarrhea. The sick child is fed often. Digestive power is practically absent. The additional food given ferments and more serum has to be thrown out to protect the intestinal walls. Soon there is a well established case of cholera infantum.

If only enough food had been given to satisfy bodily requirements, none of the milk would have spoiled in the alimentary tract. If all feeding had been stopped as soon as the child became irritable and pinched looking about the mouth and nose, and all the water desired had been given and the child kept warm, there would have been no serious disease. In these cases, the less food given the quicker the recoveries and the fewer the fatalities.

Another common disease of childhood is adenoids. To talk of these maladies as diseases is rather misleading, for they are merely symptoms of perverted nutrition, but we are compelled to make the best of our medical language.

Adenoids are due to indigestion. The indigestion is due to overeating. This is how it comes about: A child eats more than can be digested, generally bolting the food, which is often of a mushy character. The excessive amount of food can not be digested, and as the intestines and the stomach are moist and have a temperature of 100 degrees Fahrenheit, fermentation soon takes place. Some of the results of fermentation in the alimentary tract are acids, gases and bacterial poisons. These deleterious substances are absorbed into the blood stream and go to all parts of the body, acting as irritants. We do not know why they cause adenoids in one child and catarrh in another. It is easy enough to say that children are predisposed that way, which is no information at all. It seems that all of us have some weak point, and here disease has a tendency to localize. What part the sympathetic nervous system plays, we do not know. Glandular tissue is rather unstable and therefore it becomes diseased easily and adenoids are therefore quite frequent.

A coated tongue, or an irritated tongue, both due to indigestion, is a concomitant of adenoids. Such diseases do not merely happen. There are good reasons for their appearance. They are not reflections on the child, but they are on the parents who should have the right knowledge and should take time and pains enough to educate and train the child into health.

Tuberculosis is one of the results of ruined nutrition. First there is overeating. This causes indigestion. The irritating products of food fermenting in the alimentary tract are taken up by the blood. The blood goes to the lungs where it irritates the delicate mucous membrane. In self-protection it begins to secrete an excess of mucus and if the irritation is great enough, pus. The various bacteria are incidental. The tubercular bacillus is never able to gain a foothold in healthy lungs, but after degeneration of lung-tissue has taken place the lungs furnish a splendid home for this bacillus. The tubercular bacillus is a scavenger and therefore does not thrive in healthy bodies. It is the result of disease, not the cause.

Tubercular subjects never have healthy digestive organs. Unfortunately, nearly all of them are persuaded to eat many times more food than they can digest, and thus they have no opportunity to recover, for the overfeeding ruins the digestive and assimilative powers beyond recuperative ability. A large per cent. of the human race perish miserably from this disease, which results principally from the ingestion of too much food. The liberal use of such devitalized foods as sterilized milk, refined sugar and finely bolted wheat flour is doubtless a great factor in so reducing bodily resistance that the system falls an easy prey to disease. Too little breathing and poor, devitalized air are also important factors.

There are many causes of rheumatism, but overeating is the chief and it is very doubtful if a case of rheumatism can develop without this main cause. Exposure is often given as the cause, but a healthy man with a clean body does not become rheumatic.

Rheumatism is due to internal filth. A filthy alimentary tract makes filthy blood. Some say that the poison in rheumatism is uric acid, and perhaps it is, but there are no uric acid deposits in the body of a prudent eater. The elimination in this disease is imperfect. The skin, the kidneys, the bowels and the lungs do not throw out the debris as they should. Perhaps only one or two of these organs are acting inadequately. The debris is stored up in the system.

Why do the organs of elimination fail to act? Because so much work is thrust upon them that they grow weary and worn; also, a part of the material furnished them is the product of decay in the alimentary tract, and they can not thrive on poor material. Too much food is eaten. An excess of nutritive material, poorly digested, is absorbed. And so we come back to the principal cause, overeating.

When the eliminative organs fail to perform their function, the waste is deposited in those parts of the body which are weakened. The irritation from these foreign substances causes inflammation and the result is pain. The extent to which this depositing of material will go is well illustrated in some cases of multiple articular rheumatism, or arthritis deformans, where the deposits are so great that many of the joints become fixed (anchylosed).

We could review all the diseases, and nearly every time we would come back to disturbed nutrition as the principal factor, and this is true of not only physical ills, but the mental ones as well.

Various foods do not combine well, still if they are eaten in moderation they do but little harm. If we overeat, the evil results are bound to manifest, no matter how good the food, though it sometimes takes years before they are perceptible. The effects are cumulative. Each day there is a little fermentation with absorption of the poisonous products. Each day the body degenerates a little. The time always comes when the body can continue its work no longer, and then the individual must choose between reform on one hand and suffering or death on the other.

It is very difficult to convince people that they eat too much. Indeed, the average person is a small eater, in his own estimation. We have been educated into consuming such vast quantities of food that we hardly know what moderation is. In the past, physiologists and observers have watched the amount of food that people could coax down and this they have called the normal amount of food. This is far from the truth. The average American eats at least two times as much as he can digest, assimilate and use to advantage. Many eat three and four times too much. However, nature is very tolerant for a while. Most of us start out with a fair amount of resistance and are thus enabled to live to the age of forty or fifty in spite of abuses. If we could only dispense with our excesses, we could double or treble our life span, live better, get more enjoyment out of life and give the world more and better work than we can under present conditions.

There is much talk of food shortage. The amount of food consumed and wasted annually in the United States is enough to feed 200,000,000 people. Even with our present knowledge we can easily produce twice as much per acre as we are averaging, and we are tilling only about one-fourth of the land that could be made productive. If we use our brains there is little danger of starving. What is needed now is not more food, but intelligent distribution and consumption of what we produce.

We hear of cases of undernourishment. This doubtless occurs at times in the congested parts of great centers of populations. But there are not so many cases suffering from want of the proper quantity of food as from want of quality of food. Bread of finely bolted white flour is starvation food, no matter how great the quantity, unless other food rich in organic salts is also eaten.

The overeating habit is so common and comes on so insidiously that the sufferers do not realize that they are eating to excess. The resultant discomforts are blamed on other things. Babies are fed every two hours or oftener. They should be fed but three or at most four times a day, and never at night. When able to eat solid foods they get three meals a day and generally two or more lunches. Some children seem to be lunching at all times. They have fruit or bread and butter with jelly or jam in the hand almost all the time. They are encouraged to eat much and often to produce growth and strength. This kind of feeding often does produce large children, heavy in weight, but they are not healthy. Sad to relate, the excess causes disease and death.

Such frequent feeding allows the digestive organs no rest. The overwork imposed upon them and the fermentation cause irritation. This irritation manifests in a constant and almost irresistible desire for food, as does the consumption of much alcohol cause a desire for more alcohol, as the use of morphine or cocaine produces a dominating and ruinous appetite for more of these drugs. These appetites grow by what they feed upon. Man ceases to be master and becomes the abject slave of his abnormal cravings.

Slaves of alcohol and the various habit-forming drugs generally lack the strength of body and mind to assert themselves and to regain mastery of themselves. Coffee and tea have their victims, though they are generally not very firmly enslaved. No one realizes how he is bound by his cravings for an excessive amount of food until he tries to break the bonds. Such people may eat moderately for days, perhaps for weeks, and then the old appetite reasserts itself in all its strength and unless the sufferer has a very strong will a food debauch follows. I have seen men go from one restaurant to another, consuming enormous quantities of food to efface the awful craving, just as men go from one saloon to another to satisfy their desire for alcohol. The gluttons often look with the greatest contempt upon the slaves of liquor. But what is the difference? No matter what appetite, what habit, what passion has gained the mastery, we are slaves. The important thing is to keep out of slavery, or break the bonds and regain freedom.

Those who eat to excess often eat more than three times a day. They take a little candy now, a little fruit then, or they go to the drug store for a glass of malted milk or buttermilk, which they call drinks, or they take a dish of ice cream. The housewife nibbles at cake or bread. If a person is in fair health and wishes to evolve into self-mastery and good health, he should make up his mind never to eat more than three times a day. Nothing but plain water should enter his mouth except at meal times.

Next he should limit the number of articles eaten at a meal. The breakfast and lunch should each consist of no more than two or three varieties of food. The dinner should not exceed five or six varieties, and if that many are eaten, they should be compatible. Less would be be better. The less variety we have, the better the food digests. Also, eating ten or twelve or more kinds of food, as many people do, always leads to overeating. A little of this added to a little of that soon makes a too great total. It is easy to eat all one should of a certain article of food and feel satisfied, and then change off to something else and before one is through one has eaten three or four times as much as necessary. If the meal is to consist of starch there is no great objection to a small amount of bread, potatoes, rice, macaroni and chestnuts. However, a normal person does not need to coax food down by using great variety. Those who mix their foods this way invariably overeat. Besides, the various starches require different periods for digestion. Rice is more easily disposed of than bread. Each new item stimulates the desire for more food. It is best, when having potatoes, to have no other starchy food in that meal; or when bread is eaten, to have no potatoes or other starchy food. The habit of eating meat, potatoes and bread in the same meal is very common and causes much disease.

Next the searcher for health should teach himself to eat foods that are natural, cooked simply, and with a minimum amount of seasoning and dressing. The various spices and sauces irritate the digestive organs and create a craving for an excessive amount of food. The food should be changed as little as possible because such denatured foods as white flour, polished rice, pasteurized milk, and many of the canned fruits and vegetables are so lacking in the natural salts that they do not satisfy one's desire for organic salts. Overeating results.

Preserves, jellies and jams are open to the same objection. They cause an abnormal desire for food. Therefore, they should be used seldom and very sparingly. So long as apples, oranges, figs, dates, raisins, sweet prunes and various other fruits can be had, there is no excuse for the consumption of great quantities of the heavily sugared concoctions which are now so popular.

Simplicity and naturalness are great aids in breaking away from food slavery. They are discussed more fully elsewhere. In the next chapter will be found hints on the solution of the normal amount of food to be eaten.

CHAPTER V.

DAILY FOOD INTAKE.

It is generally believed that the more we eat the better. Physicians say that it is necessary to eat heartily when well to retain health and strength. When ill it is necessary to consume much food to regain lost health and strength. "Eat all you can of nourishing food," is a common free prescription, and it sounds very reasonable. The physicians of today are not to blame for this belief in overeating, for they were taught thus at college, and very few men in any line do original thinking. It has been a racial belief for centuries and no one now living is responsible. When a physician advocates what he honestly believes he is doing his best, "and angels can do no more."

When a child loses its appetite, the parents worry, for they think that it is very harmful for young people to go without food for a few meals. A lost appetite is nature's signal to quit eating, and it should always be heeded. If it is, it will prevent much disease and suffering and will save many lives.

The present-day mode of preparing food leads to overeating. The sense of taste is ruined by the stimulants put into the food. Dishes are so numerous and so temptingly made that more is eaten than can be digested and assimilated. Refined sugar, salt, the various spices, pickles, sauces and preserves all lead to overeating because of stimulation. The same is true of alcohol taken immediately before meals. If we only give nature a chance, and are perfectly frank and honest with ourselves, she will guard us against the overconsumption of food. Those who eat but few varieties of plain food at a meal are not sorely tempted to overeat. But when one savory dish is served after another it takes much will power to be moderate.

People generally have had more than sufficient before the last course is served. However, the various dishes have different flavors and for this reason the palate is overwhelmed and accepts more food than is good for us.

Men who like to call their work scientific, figure on the amount of food we need to furnish a certain number of heat units--calories. Heat, of course, is a form of energy. Basing the body's food requirements on heat units expended does not solve the problem. The more food that is ingested, the more heat units must be manufactured, and often so much food is taken that the body is compelled to go into the heating business. Then we have fevers.

A large part of the heat is given off by the skin. Those who overeat are compelled to do a great deal of radiating. This excessive amount of fuel taken into the system in the form of food, wears out the body. As figured by the experts, it gives a result of food need that is at least twice as great as necessary. Experience is the only correct guide to food requirements, and each individual has to settle the matter for himself. The human body is not exactly a chemical laboratory, nor is it an engine which can be fed so much fuel with the resultant production of such and such an amount of heat and energy. Some bodies are more efficient than others. It is among human beings as among the lower animals, some require more food than others.

We need enough food to repair the waste, to perform our work and to furnish heat. Every muscle contraction uses up a little energy. Every breath deprives us of heat and carries away carbon dioxide, the latter being formed by oxidation of tissues in the body. Every minute we lose heat by radiation from the skin. Every thought requires a small amount of food. If we worry, the leak of nervous energy is tremendous, but at the same time we put ourselves in position where we are unable to replenish our stock, for worry ruins digestion. All this expenditure of energy and loss of heat must be made up for by the food intake. Only a small amount of surplus food can be stored in the body. Some fat can be stored as fat. Some starch and sugar can be put aside as either glycogen--animal sugar--or be changed into fat. This storing of excess food is very limited, except in cases of obesity, which is a disease.

Overeating invariably causes disease. It may take two or three years, yes even twenty or thirty years, before the overeating results in serious illness, but the results are certain, and in the meanwhile the individual is never up to par. He can use neither body nor mind to the best advantage.

To emphasize and illustrate these remarks, I shall copy a few diet lists, which their authors consider reasonable and correct for the average person for one day, and I shall give my comments. The first is taken from Kirke's Physiology, which has been used extensively as a text-book in medical colleges:

340 grams lean uncooked meat, 600 " bread, 90 " butter, 28 " cheese, 225 " potatoes, 225 " carrots.

An ounce contains 28.3 grams; a pound, 453 grams. It is easy to figure these quantities of food in ounces or pounds, which give a better idea to the average person.

It is self-evident that this is too much food. Over twelve ounces of lean, uncooked meat, over twenty-one ounces of bread, almost one-half of a pound each of potatoes and carrots, about an ounce of cheese and over three ounces of butter make enough food for two days, even for a big eater. He who tries to live up to a diet of this kind is sure to suffer disease and early death.

The average loaf of bread weighs about fourteen ounces. Here we are told to devour one-half of a pound of carrots (for which other vegetables such as turnips, parsnips, beets or cabbage may be substituted), one-half of a pound of potatoes, three-fourths of a pound of lean raw meat, which loses some weight in cooking, a loaf and one-half of bread, besides butter and cheese. The vast majority of people can not eat more than one-third of this amount and retain efficiency and health, but many eat even more.

The next table is taken from Dr. I. Burney Yeo's book on diet, and is given as the food required daily by a "well nourished worker":

151.3 grams meat, 48.1 " white of egg, 450.0 " bread, 500.0 " milk, 1065.9 " beer, 60.2 " suet, 30.0 " butter, 70.0 " starch, 17.0 " sugar, 4.9 " salt.

This worker is too well fed. Often those who are so well fed are poorly nourished, for the excessive amount of food ruins the nutrition, after which the food is poorly digested and assimilated. This worker eats so much that he will be compelled to do manual labor all his days, for such feeding prevents effective thinking.

The following daily average diet is taken from the book, "Diet and Dietetics," by A. Gauthier, a well known authority on the subject of the nutritive needs of the body. Mr. Gauthier averaged the daily food intake of the inhabitants of Paris for the ten years from 1890 to 1899, inclusive. He takes it for granted that this is the average daily food requirement for a person:

420.0 grams bread and cakes, 216.0 " boned meat, 24.1 " eggs (weighed with shell), 8.1 " cheese (dry or cream), 28.0 " butter, oil, etc., 70.0 " fresh fruit, 250.0 " green vegetables, 40.0 " dried vegetables, 100.0 " potatoes, rice, 40.0 " sugar, 20.0 " salt, 213.0 C. C. milk, 557.0 C. C. of various alcoholics, containing 9.5 C. C. of pure alcohol.

So long as the Parisians consume such quantities of food they will continue to suffer and die before they reach one-half of the age that should be theirs. The French eat no more than do other people, in fact, they seem moderate in their food intake as compared with some of the Germans, English and Americans, but they eat too much for their physical and mental good.

The lists given above are from sources that command the respect of the medical profession. They are the orthodox and popular opinions. It would be an easy matter to give many more tables, but they agree so closely that it would be a waste of time and space.

Quantitative tables from vegetarian sources are not so common. The vegetarians say that meat eating is wrong, being contrary to nature. Whether they are right or wrong, they make the same mistakes that the orthodox prescribers do, that is, they advocate overeating. Medical textbooks prescribe a too abundant supply of starch and meat in particular. The vegetarians prescribe a superabundance of starch. Read the magazines advocating vegetarianism and note their menus, giving numerous cereals, tubers, peas, beans, lentils, as well as other vegetables, for the same meal. It is as easy to overeat of nuts and protein in leguminous vegetables as it is to overeat of meat.

Starch poisoning is as bad as meat poisoning and the results are equally fatal.

The following are suggestions offered by a fruitarian. They give the food intake for two days:

120 grams shelled peanuts, raw, 1000 " apples, 500 " unfermented whole wheat bread.

120 grams shelled filberts, 450 " raisins, 800 " bananas.

In the first day's menu it will be noted that over two pounds of apples and over one pound of whole wheat bread are recommended, also over four ounces of raw peanuts. The writer says that this food should preferably be taken in two meals. There are very few people with enough digestive and assimilative power to care for more than one-half of a pound of whole wheat bread twice a day, especially when taken with raw peanuts, which are rather hard to digest. The trouble is made worse by the addition of more than one pound of apples to each meal, for when apples in large quantities are eaten with liberal amounts of starch, the tendency for the food to ferment is so strong that only a very few escape. Gas is produced in great quantities, which is both unnatural and unpleasant. Neither stomach nor bowels manufacture any perceptible amount of gas if they are in good condition and a moderate amount of food is taken.

Whole wheat bread digests easily enough when eaten in moderation, but it is very difficult to digest when as much as eight ounces are taken at a meal. One can accustom the body to accept this amount of food, but it is never required under ordinary conditions and the results in the long run are bad.

The food prescribed for the second day is more easily digested, but it is too much. Raisins are a splendid force food, but no ordinary individual needs a pound of raisins in one day, in addition to about one and three-fourths pounds of bananas, which are also a force food and are about as nourishing as the same amount of Irish potatoes.

In all my reading it has not been my good fortune to find a diet table for healthy people, giving moderate quantities of food. Diet lists seem scientific, so they appeal to the mind that has not learned to think of the subject from the correct point of view. Quantitative diet tables are worthless, for one person may need more than another. Some are short and some are tall. Some are naturally slender and others of stocky build. There is as much difference in people's food needs as there is in their appearance. To try to fit the same quantity and even kind of food to all is as senseless as it would be to dress all in garments of identical size and cut.

If we eat in moderation it does not make much difference what we eat, provided our diet contains either raw fruits or raw vegetables enough to furnish the various mineral salts and the food is fairly well prepared. There are combinations that are not ideal, but they do very little harm if there is no overeating. People who are moderate in their eating generally relish simple foods. Unfortunately, there is but little moderation in eating. From childhood on the suggestion that it is necessary to eat liberally is ever before us. Medical men, grandparents, parents and neighbors think and talk alike. If the parents believe in moderation, the neighbors kindly give lunches to the children. It is really difficult to raise children right, especially in towns and cities.

After such training we learn to believe in overeating and we pass the belief on to the next generation, as it has in the past been handed down from generation to generation. Finally we die, many of us martyrs to overconsumption of food. Ask any healer of intelligence who has thrown off the blinders put on at college and who has allowed himself to think without fear, and he will tell you that at least nine-tenths of our ills come from improper eating habits. It is not difficult to make up menus of compatible foods. No one knows how much another should eat, and he who prepares quantitative diet tables for the multitude must fail.

However, every individual of ordinary intelligence can quickly learn his own food requirements and the key thereto is given by nature. It is not well to think of one's self much or often. It is not well to be introspective, but everyone should get acquainted with himself, learning to know himself well enough to treat himself with due consideration. We are taught kindness to others. We need to be taught kindness to ourselves. The average person ought to be able to learn his normal food requirements within three or four months, and a shorter time will often suffice.

The following observations will prove helpful to the careful reader:

Food should have a pleasant taste while it is being eaten, but should not taste afterwards. If it does it is a sign of indigestion following overeating, or else it indicates improper combinations or very poor cooking. Perhaps food was taken when there was no desire for it, which is always a mistake. Perhaps too many foods were combined in the meal. Or it may be that there was not enough mouth preparation. It is generally due to overeating. Cabbage, onions, cucumbers and various other foods which often repeat, will not do so when properly prepared and eaten in moderation, if other conditions are right.

Eructation of gas and gas in the bowels are indications of overeating. More food is taken than can be digested. A part of it ferments and gas is a product of fermentation. A very small amount of gas in the alimentary tract is natural, but when there is belching or rumbling of gas in the intestines it is a sign of indigestion, which may be so mild that the individual is not aware of it, or it may be so bad that he can think of little else. When there is formation of much gas it is always necessary to reduce the food intake, and to give special attention to the mastication of all starch-containing aliments. Also, if starches and sour fruits have been combined habitually, this combination should be given up. Starch digests in an alkaline medium, and if it is taken with much acid by those whose digestive powers are weak, the result is fermentation instead of digestion.

People should never eat enough to experience a feeling of languor. They should quit eating before they feel full. If there is a desire to sleep after meals, too much food has been ingested. When drowsiness possesses us after meals we have eaten so much that the digestive organs require so much blood that there is not enough left for the brain. This is a hint that if we have work or study that requires exceptional clearness of mind, we should eat very moderately or not at all immediately before. The digestive organs appropriate the needed amount of blood and the brain refuses to do its best when deprived of its normal supply of oxygen and nourishment.

Serpents, some beasts of prey and savages devour such large quantities of food at times that they go into a stupor. There is no excuse for our patterning after them now that a supply of food is easily obtained at all times.

A bad taste in the mouth is usually a sign of overeating. It comes from the decomposition following a too liberal food intake. If water has a bad taste in the morning or at any other time, it indicates overeating. It may be due to a filthy mouth or the use of alcohol.

Heartburn is also due to overeating, and so is hiccough; both come from fermentation of food in the alimentary tract.

A heavily coated tongue in the morning indicates excessive food intake. If the tongue is what is known as a dirty gray color it shows that the owner has been overeating for years. The normal mucous membrane is clean and pink. The mucous membrane of the mouth, stomach and the first part of the bowels should not be compelled to act as an organ of excretion, for the normal function is secretory and absorptive. However, when so much food is eaten that the skin, lungs, kidneys and lower bowel can not throw off all the waste and excess, the mucous membrane in the upper part of the alimentary tract must assist. The result is a coated tongue, but the tongue is in no worse condition than the mucous membrane of the stomach. A coated tongue indicates overcrowded nutrition and is nature's request to reduce the food intake. How much? Enough to clean the tongue. If the coating is chronic it may take several months before the tongue becomes clean.

A muddy skin, perhaps pimply, is another sign of overeating. It shows that the food intake is so great that the body tries to eliminate too many of the solids through the skin, which becomes irritated from this cause and the too acid state of the system and then there is inflammation. Many forms of eczema and a great many other skin diseases are caused by stomach disorders and an overcrowded nutrition. There is a limit to the skin's excretory ability, and when this is exceeded skin diseases ensue. Some of the so-called incurable skin diseases get well in a short time on a proper diet without any local treatment.

Dull eyes and a greenish tinge of the whites of the eyes point toward digestive disturbances due to an oversupply of food. The green color comes from bile thrown into the blood when the liver is overworked. The liver is never overtaxed unless the consumption of food is excessive.

Another very common sign of too generous feeding is catarrh, and it does not matter where the catarrh is located. It is true that there are other causes of catarrh, in fact, anything that irritates the mucous membrane any length of time will cause it, but an overcrowded nutrition causes the ordinary cases. It is the same old story: The mucous membrane is forced to take on the function of eliminating superfluous matter, which has been taken into the system in the form of food. Many people dedicate their lives to the act of turning a superabundance of food into waste, and as a result they overwork their bodies so that they are never well physically and seldom efficient mentally.

Many people, especially women, say that if they miss a meal or get it later than usual, they suffer from headache. This indicates that the feeding is wrong, generally too generous and often too stimulating. A normal person can miss a dozen meals without a sign of a headache.

To repeat: No one can tell how much another should eat, but everyone can learn for himself what the proper amount of food is. Enough is given above to help solve the problem. The interpretations presented are not the popular ones, but they are true for they give good results when acted upon.

If bad results follow a meal there has been overeating, either at the last meal or previously. Undermasticating usually accompanies overeating and causes further trouble. Those who masticate thoroughly are generally quite moderate in their food intake.

Many say that they eat so much because they enjoy their food so. He who eats too rapidly or in excess does not know what true enjoyment of food is. Excessive eating causes food poisoning, and food poisoning blunts all the special senses. To have normal smell, taste, hearing and vision one must be clean through and through, and those who are surfeited with food are not clean internally.

The average individual does not know the natural taste of most foods. He seasons them so highly that the normal taste is hidden or destroyed. Those who wish to know the exquisite flavor of such common foods as onions, carrots, cabbage, apples and oranges must eat them without seasoning or dressing for a while. To get real enjoyment from food it is necessary to eat slowly and in moderation.

I know both from personal experience and from the experience of others that seasoning is not necessary. Instead of giving the foods better flavor, they taste inferior. A little salt will harm no one, but the constant use of much seasoning leads to irritation of the digestive organs and to overeating. Salt taken in excess also helps to bring on premature aging. It is splendid for pickling and preserving, but health and life in abundance are the only preservatives needed for the body. Refined sugar should be classed among the condiments. People who live normally lose the desire for it. Grapefruit, for instance, tastes better when eaten plain than when sugar is added.

People who sleep seven or eight hours and wake up feeling unrefreshed are suffering from the ingestion of too much food. A food poisoned individual can not be properly rested. To get sweet sleep and feel restored it is necessary to have clean blood and a sweet alimentary tract.

Much has been said about overeating. Once in a while a person will habitually undereat, but such cases are exceedingly rare. To undereat is foolish. At all times we must use good sense. It is a subject upon which no fixed rules can be promulgated. Be guided by the feelings, for perfect health is impossible to those who lack balance.

Those who think they need scientific direction may take one of the orthodox diet tables. If it contains alcoholics, remove them from the list. Then partake of about one-third of the starch recommended, and about one-third of the protein. Use more fresh fruit and fresh vegetables than listed. Instead of eating bread made from white flour, use whole wheat bread. Do not try to eat everything given on the scientific diet list each day. For instance, rice, potatoes and bread are given in many of these tables. Select one of these starches one day, another the next day, etc. If one-third of the amount recommended is too much, and it sometimes is, reduce still further.

Please bear in mind that the orthodox way, the so-called scientific way, has been tried over a long period of time and it has given very poor results. Moderation has always given good results and always will.

CHAPTER VI.

WHAT TO EAT.

It is very important to eat the right kind of food, but it is even more important to be balanced and use common sense. Those who are moderate in their habits and cheerful can eat almost anything with good results. Of course, people who live almost entirely on such denatured foods as polished rice, finely bolted wheat flour products, sterilized milk and meat spoiled in the cooking, refined sugar and potatoes deprived of most of their salts through being soaked and cooked will suffer.

There are many different diet systems, and some of them are very good. If their advocates say that their way is the only way, they are wrong. Many try to force their ideas upon others. They find their happiness in making others miserable. They are afflicted with the proselyting zeal that makes fools of people. This is the wrong way to solve the food problem. Let each individual choose his own way and allow those who differ to continue in the old way.

Many have changed their dietary habits to their own great benefit. After this they become so enthused and anxious for others to do likewise that they wear themselves and others out exhorting them to share in the new discovery. This does no good, but it often does harm, for it leads the zealot to think too much of and about himself, and it annoys others.

Many are like my friend who lunched daily on zwieback and raw carrots. "I think everybody ought to eat some raw carrots every day; don't you?" she said. We can not mold everybody to our liking, and we should not try. If we conquer ourselves, we have about all we can do. If we succeed in this great work, we will evolve enough tolerance to be willing to allow others to shape their own ends. To volunteer undesired information does no good, for it creates opposition in the mind of the hearers. If the information is sought, the chances are that it may in time do good. It is well enough to indicate how and where better knowledge may be obtained. We should at all times attempt to conserve our energy and use it only when and where it is helpful. Such conduct leads to peace of mind, effectiveness, happiness and health.

The tendency to become too enthusiastic about a dietary regime that has brought personal benefit is to be avoided, for it brings unnecessary odium upon the important subject of food reform. People do not like to change old habits, even if the change would be for the better, and when an enthusiast tries to force the change his actions are resented. He makes no real converts, but as pay for his efforts he gains the reputation of being a crank.

Those who wish to be helpful in an educational way should be patient. The race has been in the making for ages. Its good habits, as well as its bad ones, have been acquired gradually. If we ever get rid of our bad habits it will be through gradual evolution, not through a hasty revolution. We need a change in dietary habits, but those who become food cranks, insisting that others be as they, retard this movement. Only a few will change physical and mental habits suddenly. If those who know are content to show the benefits more in results than in words, their influence for good will be great.

What shall we eat? How are we to know the truth among so many conflicting ideas? We can know the truth because it leads to health. Error leads to suffering, degeneration and premature death. As the homely saying goes, "The proof of the pudding is in the eating."

Let us look into some of the diet theories before the public and give them thoughtful consideration.

The late Dr. J. H. Salisbury advocated the use of water to drink and meat to eat, and nothing else. The water was to be taken warm and in copious quantities, but not at or near meal time. The meat, preferably beef, was to be scraped or minced, made into cakes and cooked in a very warm skillet until the cakes turned gray within. These meat cakes were to be eaten three times a day, seasoned with salt and a little pepper.

The doctor had a very successful practice, which is attested by many who were benefited when ordinary medical skill failed. His diet was not well balanced. In meats there is a lack of the cell salts and force food. Especially are the cell salts lacking when the flesh is drained of its blood. The animals of prey drink the blood and crunch many of the bones of their victims, thus getting nearly all the salts. But in spite of his giving such an unbalanced diet, the doctor had a satisfactory practice and good success. Why? Because his patients had to quit using narcotics and stimulants and they were compelled to consume such simple food that they ceased overeating. It is a well known fact that a mono-diet forces moderation, for there is no desire to overeat, as there is when living on a very varied diet.

Another fact that the Salisbury plan brings to mind is that starch and sugar are not necessary for the feeding of adults, although they are convenient and cheap foods and ordinarily consumed in large quantities. The fat in the meat takes the place of the starch and sugar. Atomically, starch, sugar and fat are almost identical, and they can be substituted one for the other. Nature makes broad provisions.

Dr. Salisbury's career also serves to remind us that a mixed diet is not necessary for the physical welfare of those who eat to live. Vegetarians dwell upon the toxicity of meat. But Dr. Salisbury fed his patients on nothing but meat and water, and the percentage of recoveries in chronic diseases was considered remarkable. Meat is very easy to digest and when prepared in the simple manner prescribed by the doctor and eaten by itself it will agree with nearly everybody. But when eaten with soup, bread, potatoes, vegetables, cooked and raw, fish, pudding, fruit, coffee, crackers and cheese, there will be overeating followed by indigestion and its consequent train of ills. However, it is not fair to blame the meat entirely, for the whole mixture goes into decomposition and poisons the body.

The cures resulting from Dr. Salisbury's plan also help to disprove the much heralded theory of Dr. Haig, that uric acid from meat eating is the cause of rheumatism. Overeating of meat is often a contributory cause. We are told that the rheumatics who followed Dr. Salisbury's plan got well. They regained physical tone. They lost their gout and rheumatism. They parted company with their pimples and blotches. All of which would indicate that the blood became clean.

The chief lesson derived from Dr. Salisbury's plan and experience is the helpfulness of simple living and moderation. An exclusive diet of meat is not well balanced. Energy produced from flesh food is too expensive. The good results came from substituting habits of simplicity and moderation for the habit of overeating of too great variety of food. The same results may be obtained by putting a patient on bread and milk.

Dr. Salisbury's patients had unsatisfied longings, doubtless for various tissue salts. The addition of fresh raw fruits or vegetables would improve his diet, for apples, peaches, pears, lettuce, celery and cabbage are rich in the salts in which meats are deficient.

Dr. Emmet Densmore recommended omitting the starches entirely, that is, to avoid such foods as cereals, tubers and legumes. He believed that it is best to live on fruits and nuts. He recommended the sweet fruits--figs, dates, raisins, prunes--instead of the starchy foods. The doctor did much good, as everyone does who gets his patients to simplify. He also had good results before discovering that starch is a harmful food, when he fed his patients bread and milk.

Starch must be converted into sugar before it can be used by the body. The sugar is what is known as dextrose, not the refined sugar of commerce. The sweet fruits contain this sugar in the form of fruit sugar, which needs but little preparation to be absorbed by the blood. Dr. Densmore reasons thus: Only birds are furnished with mills (gizzards); hence the grains are fit food for them only. Other starches should be avoided because they are difficult to digest, the doctor wrote.

Raw starches are difficult to digest, but when they are properly cooked they are digested in a reasonable time without overburdening the system, provided they are well masticated and the amount eaten is not too great and the combining is correct. Rice, which contains much starch, digests in a short time.

We can do very nicely without starch. We can also thrive on it if we do not abuse it. The two chief starch-bearing staples, rice and wheat, contain considerable protein and salts in their natural state. In fact, the natural wheat will sustain life for a long time. Man has improved on nature by polishing the rice and making finely bolted, bleached wheat flour, deprived of nearly all the salts in the wheat berry. The result is that both of them have become very poor foods. The more we eat of these refined products the worse off we are, unless we partake freely of other foods rich in mineral salts.

Not long ago a lady died in England who was a prominent advocate of a "brainy diet." Her brainy diet consisted largely of excessive quantities of meat, pork being a favorite. She died comparatively young, her friends say from overwork. Such a diet doubtless had a large part in wearing her out. To overeat of meat is dangerous.

A gentleman is now advocating a diet of nothing but cocoanuts. This is a fad, for they are not a balanced food. He has published a book on the subject. Perhaps his advocacy is influenced by his interest in the sale of cocoanuts.

The vegetarians condemn the use of meat. Some of them are called fruitarians. It is very difficult to decide who are the most representative of them. Some advocate the use of nothing but fruit and nuts. Others add cereals to this. Others use vegetables in addition. Some even allow the use of dairy products and eggs, that is, all foods except flesh.

They say that meat is an unnatural food for man and condemn its use on moral grounds. It is difficult to decide what is natural, for we find that man is very adaptable, being able to live on fruits in the tropics and almost exclusively on flesh food, largely fat, in the arctic regions. In nature the strong live on the weak and the intelligent on the dull. There is no sentiment in nature. In her domain might, physical or mental, makes right. Sentiments of right and justice are not highly developed except among human beings, and even there they are so weakly implanted that it takes but little provocation for civilized man to bare his teeth in a wolfish snarl.

With some vegetarianism is largely a matter of esthetics, ethics and morality. Morality is based on expediency, so it really is a question whether meat is an advantageous food or not.

Another vegetarian argument is that man's anatomy proves that he was not intended by nature to eat meat. Good arguments have been used on both sides, but they are not very convincing nor are they conclusive. It is hard to draw any lines fairly.

Another objection to meat is that it is unclean and full of poisons, that these poisons produce various diseases, such as cancer. We are also informed that refined sugar causes cancer, and the belief in tomatoes as a causative factor is not dead. Cancer is without doubt caused principally by dietary indiscretions but it is impossible to single out any one food.

No matter what foods we eat, we are compelled to be careful or they will be unclean. Those who wish clean meat can obtain it. The amount of poison or waste in a proper portion of meat is so small that we need give it no thought.

Those who eat in moderation can take meat once a day during cold weather and enjoy splendid health. During warm weather it should be eaten more seldom.

On the other hand, meat is not necessary. We need a certain amount of protein, which we can obtain from nuts, eggs, milk, cheese, peanuts, peas, beans, lentils, cereals and from other food in smaller amounts. The amount of protein needed is small--about one-fifth of what the physiologists used to recommend.

Those who think meat eating is wrong should not partake of it. They can get along very well without it. We are consuming entirely too much meat in America. The organism can stand it if the life is active in the fresh air, but it will not do for people who are housed. Much meat eating causes physical degeneration. The body loses tone. Experiments have shown that vegetarians have more resistance and endurance than the meat eaters, but the meat eaters get so much stimulation from their food that they can speed up in spurts. The excretions of meat eaters are more poisonous than those of vegetarians.

Eggs produced by hens fed largely on meat scraps do not keep as well as those laid by hens feeding more on grains. In short, meat eating leads to instability or degeneration, if carried to excess. Young children should have none of it and it would be a very easy matter for the rising generation to develop without using meat, and I believe this would be better than our present plan of eating. However, let us give flesh food the credit due it. When meat eaters are debilitated no other food seems to act as kindly as meat, given with fruits or vegetables. When properly prepared and taken in moderation meat digests easily and is quite completely assimilated.

Many make the mistake of living too exclusively on starch and taking it in excess. The result is fermentation and an acid state of the alimentary tract. Dr. Daniel S. Sager says that, "About all that we have to fear in eating is excessive use of proteids." Experience and observation do not bear out this statement, for it is as easy to find people injured by starch as by protein. One form of poisoning is as bad as the other. The doctor also warns against nearly all the succulent vegetables, saying that on account of the indigestible fibre, most of them are unfit for human consumption.

Dr. E. H. Dewey condemned the apple as a disease-producer, and inferentially, other fruits.

Dr. Charles E. Page objects to the use of milk by adults, on the ground that it is fit food only for the calves for whom nature intended it. Many writers have repeated this opinion.

Most of the regular physicians have a very vague idea of dietetics and proper feeding. When asked what to eat they commonly say, "Eat plenty nourishing food of the kinds that agree with you." They do not point out the fundamentals to their patients. Sometimes they advise avoiding combinations of milk and fruits. Sometimes they say that all starches should be avoided and in the next breath prescribe toast, one of the starchiest of foods. At times they proscribe pork and pickles but they are seldom able to give a good diet prescription. What people need is a fair knowledge of what to do and the don'ts will take care of themselves.

All foods have been condemned as unfit for human consumption by people who should know. However, those who look at these matters with open eyes and open minds will come to the conclusion that man is a very adaptable animal; that if necessary he can get along without almost all foods, being able to subsist on a very small variety; that he can live for a long period on animal food entirely; that he can live all his life without tasting flesh; that he can live on a mixed diet; that he can adopt a great many plans of eating and live in health and comfort on nearly all of them, provided he does not deprive himself of the natural salts and gets some protein; and finally and most important, that moderation is the chief factor in keeping well, for the best foods produce disease in time if taken in excess.

Those who object to flesh, dairy products, cereals, tubers, legumes, refined sugars, fruits or vegetables, should do without the class which they find objectionable, for it is easy to substitute from other classes. Eggs, milk or legumes may be taken in place of flesh foods. The salts contained in fruits may be obtained from vegetables. The starch, which is the chief ingredient of cereals, is easily obtained from tubers and legumes; fats and sugars will take its place. Commercial sugar is not a necessity. The force and heat derived from it can be obtained from starches and fats.

Outside of milk in infancy, there is not a single indispensable food. Some people have peculiarities which prevent them from eating certain foods, such as pork, eggs, milk and strawberries, but with these exceptions a healthy person can eat any food he pleases, provided he is moderate. We eat too much flesh, sugar and starch and we suffer for it. This does not prove that these foods are harmful, but that overeating is.

Sometimes the food question becomes a very trying one in the home. One individual has learned the fact that good results are obtained by using good sense and judgment in combining and consuming food, and he tries to force others to do as he does. This is unfortunate, for most people object to such actions, and though the intention is good, it accomplishes nothing, but prejudices others against sensible living. The best way is to do right yourself and let others sin against themselves and suffer until they are weary. Then, seeing how you got out of your trouble, perhaps they will come to you and accept what you have to offer.

The attempt to force people to be good or to be healthy is merely wasted effort.

The chapter devoted to Menus gives definite information regarding the proper manner in which to combine foods and arrange meals. Such information is also given in treating of the different classes of food.

CHAPTER VII.

WHEN TO EAT.

Three meals a day is the common plan. This is a matter of habit. Three meals a day are sufficient and should not be exceeded by man, woman or child. Lunching or "piecing" should never be indulged in. Children who are fed on plain, nutritious foods that contain the necessary food elements do not need lunches. Lunching is also a matter of habit, and we can safely say that it is a bad habit.

If three meals a day are taken, two should be light. He who wishes to work efficiently can not eat three hearty meals a day. If it is brain work, the digestive organs will take so much of the blood supply that an insufficient amount of blood will be left to nourish the brain. The worker feels the lack of energy. He is not inclined to do thorough work, that is, to go to the root of matters, and he therefore does indifferent work. One rule to which there is no exception is that the brain can not do its best when the digestive organs are working hard. If there is a piece of work to be done or a problem to be solved that requires all of one's powers it is best to tackle it with an empty stomach, or after a very light meal.

If the work is physical, it is not necessary to draw the line so fine. But it is well to remember that hard physical work prevents digestion. All experiments prove this. So if the labor is very trying, the eating should be light. Those who eat much because they work hard will soon wear themselves out, for hard work retards digestion, and with weakened digestion the more that is eaten, the less nourishment is extracted from it. Those who labor hard should take a light breakfast and the same kind of a noon meal. After the day's work is done, take a hearty meal. Those who perform hard physical labor, as well as those who work chiefly with their brains, should relax a while after the noon meal. A nap lasting ten to twenty minutes is very beneficial, but not necessary if relaxation is taken.

During sleep the activities of the body slow down. Most people who take a heavy meal and retire immediately thereafter feel uncomfortable when they wake in the morning. The reason is that the food did not digest well. It is always well to remain up at least two hours after eating a hearty meal.

Most people would be better off if they took but two meals a day. Those who have sedentary occupations need less fuel than manual laborers, and could get along very well on two meals a day. However, if moderation is practiced, no harm will come from eating three times a day.

In olden times many people lived on one meal a day. Some do so today and get along very well. It is easy to get plenty of nourishment from one meal, and it has the advantage of not taking so much time. Most of us spend too much time preparing for meals and eating. Once when it was rather inconvenient to get more meals, I lived for ten months on one meal a day. I enjoyed my food very much and was well nourished. For twelve years I have lived on two meals a day, one of them often consisting of nothing but some juicy fruit. Many others do likewise, not because they are prejudiced against three meals per day, but they find the two meal plan more convenient and very satisfactory.

Meat, potatoes and bread, with other foods, three times a day is a common combination. No ordinary mortal can live in health on such a diet. Such feeding results in discomfort and disease, and unless it is changed, in premature aging and death. The body needs only a certain amount of material. Sufficient can be taken in two meals. If three meals is the custom less food at a meal should be eaten. However, the general rule is that those who eat three meals per day eat fully as large ones as those who take only two.

As a rule, the meal times should be regular. We need a certain amount of nourishment, and it is well to take it regularly. This reduces friction, and is conducive to health, for the body is easily taught to fall into habits of regularity and works best when these are observed.

There should be a period of at least four and one-half to five hours between meals. It takes that long for the body to get a meal out of the way. Stomach digestion is but the beginning of the process, and this alone requires from two to five hours.

On the two-meal plan it makes very little difference whether the breakfast or the lunch is omitted. After going without breakfast for a week or two, one does not miss it. Miss the meal that it is the most troublesome to get. Dr. Dewey revived interest in the no-breakfast plan in this country. He considered it very beneficial. The doctor did not give credit where credit is due, for he insisted on going without breakfast. Omitting lunch or dinner accomplishes the same thing. He got his beneficial results from reducing the number of meals, and consequently the amount of food taken, but it is immaterial which meal is omitted.

Heavy breakfasts are very common in England and in our country. On the European continent they do not eat so much for breakfast, a cup of coffee and one roll being a favorite morning meal there. To eat nothing in the morning is better than to take coffee and rolls. To eat enough to steal one's brain away is a poor way to begin the day. Much better work could be done on some fruit or a glass of milk, or some cereal and butter than on eggs, steak potatoes, hot bread and coffee, which is not an uncommon breakfast.

When we consider the best time to eat, we come back to our old friend, moderation, and find that it is the best solution of the question, for if the meals are moderate we may with benefit take three meals a day, but no more, for there is not time enough during the day to digest more than three meals. However, it is not necessary to eat three times a day.

CHAPTER VIII.

HOW TO EAT.

It seems that all of us ought to know how to eat, for we have much practice; yet the individuals who know the true principles of nourishing the body are comparatively few. Very few healers are able to give full and explicit directions on this important subject. Some can give partial instructions, but we need a full working knowledge.

In one period of our racial history there were times when it was difficult to obtain food, as it is now among some savage people. Then it was without doubt customary to gorge, as it is among some savages now when they get a plenteous supply of food, especially of flesh food. Even among so-called civilized people, the distribution of food is so uneven that some are in want somewhere, nearly all the time. In parts of Russia, we are informed, the peasants go into a state of semi-hibernation during part of the winter, living on very small quantities of inferior food.

With rapid transportation and the extensive use of power-propelled machinery, famine should be unheard of in civilized countries. In our land there is a sufficient quantity of food and people seldom suffer because they have not enough, but considerable suffering is due to excessive intake and to poor quality of food. Weight for weight, white bread is not as valuable as whole wheat bread, though it contains as much starch. Measure for measure, boiled milk is inferior as a food to untreated milk, either fresh or clabbered. Such facts make it necessary for us to know how to eat.

The correct principles of taking nourishment to the best advantage have been fairly well known for a long time, and perhaps they have been fully discussed years ago by some author, but so far as I know Dr. E. H. Dewey is the first one who grouped them and gave them the prominence they deserve. He employed many pages in explaining clearly and forcibly these principles, which can be briefly stated as follows:

First, Be guided by the appetite in eating. Eat only when there is hunger.

Second, During acute illness fast, that is, live on water.

Third, Be moderate in eating.

Fourth, Masticate your food thoroughly.

Dr. J. H. Tilden teaches his patients the same in these words:

"Never eat when you feel badly.

"Never eat when you have no desire.

"Do not overeat.

"Thoroughly masticate and insalivate all your food."

Because these true dietetic principles are so important, probably being the most valuable information given in this book, let us give them enough consideration to fix them in the mind. They should be a part of every child's education. They should be so thoroughly learned that they become second nature, for if they are observed disease is practically impossible. Accidents may happen, but no serious disease can develop and certainly none of a chronic nature if these rules are observed, provided the individual gives himself half a chance in other ways. When the eating is correct, it is difficult to fall into bad habits mentally. Correct eating is a powerful aid to health. Health tends to produce proper thinking, which in turn leads the individual to proper acting.

First, Eat only when there is hunger: Hunger is of two kinds, normal and abnormal. The real or normal hunger was given us by nature to make us active enough to get food. If it were not for hunger, there would be no special incentive for the young to partake of nourishment and consequently many would die comfortably of starvation, perhaps enough to endanger the life of the race. Normal hunger asks for food, but no special kind of food. It is satisfied with anything that is clean and nourishing. It is strong enough to make a decided demand for food, but if there is no food to be had it will be satisfied for the time being with a glass of water and will cause no great inconvenience.

Abnormal hunger is entirely different. It is a very insistent craving and if it is not satisfied it produces bodily discomfort, perhaps headache. The gnawing remains and gives the victim no rest. Very often it must be pampered. It calls for beefsteak, or toast and tea, or sweets, or some other special food. If not satisfied the results may be nervousness, weakness or headache or some other disagreeable symptom.

When missing a meal or two brings discomfort, it is always a sign of a degenerating or degenerated body. A healthy person can go a day without food without any inconvenience. He feels a keen desire for food at meal times, but as soon as he has made up his mind that he is unable to get it or that he is not going to take any the hunger leaves. Normal hunger is a servant. Abnormal hunger is a hard master.

A person in good condition does not get weak from missing a few meals. One in poor physical condition does, although this is more apparent than real. In the abnormal person a part of the food is used as nourishment, but on account of the poor working of the digestive organs, a part decomposes and this acts as an irritant or a stimulant. The greater the irritation the more food is demanded. The temporary stimulation is followed by depression and then the sufferer is wretched. This depression is relieved by more food. Please note that it is relieved, not cured. The relief is only temporary.

All food stimulates, but only slightly. It is when the food decomposes that it becomes stimulating enough to cause trouble. It is well to remember that considerable alcoholic fermentation can take place in an abused alimentary tract. The stimulation obtained from too much food is very much like the stimulation derived from alcohol, tobacco or morphine. At first there is a feeling of well-being, which is followed by a miserable feeling of depression that demands food, alcohol, tobacco or morphine for relief, as the case may be, and no matter which habit is obtaining mastery, to indulge it is courting disaster. When a habit begins to assert itself strongly, break it, for later on it will be very difficult, so difficult that most people lack the will power to overcome it.

If there is abnormal hunger, reduce the food intake. Instead of eating five or six times a day, reduce the meals to two or three. It is quite common for such people to take lunches, which may consist of candies, ice cream, cakes, milk or buttermilk and various other things which most people do not look upon as real food. Take two or three meals a day, and let a large part of them be fresh vegetables and fresh fruits. Eat in moderation and the troublesome abnormal hunger will soon leave. By indulging it you increase it.

Many people get into trouble because they believe that they have to have protein, starch and fat at every meal. This is not necessary, for the blood takes up enough nourishment to last for quite a while. A supply of the various food elements once a day is sufficient, which means that protein needs be taken but once a day, starch once a day and fat once a day. Starch and fat serve the same purpose and one can be replaced by the other.

Cultivate a normal hunger, then fix two or three periods in which to take nourishment, and partake of nothing but water outside of these periods. If there is no desire for food when meal time comes, eat nothing, but drink all the water desired and wait until next meal time.

Second, During acute illness fast: This is so obviously correct that we should expect every normal individual to be guided by it. Even the lower animals know this and act accordingly.

According to this rule we should go without food when ill, but to do so is contrary to the teachings of medical men. They teach that when people are ill there is much waste, which is true, and that for this reason it is necessary to partake of a generous amount of nourishing food, so they give milk, broth, meat, toast and other foods, together with stimulants. Feeding during illness would be all right if the body could take care of the food, which it can not. In all severe diseases digestion is almost or quite at a standstill and the food given under the circumstances decomposes in the alimentary tract and furnishes additional poison for the system to excrete. Food under the circumstances is a detriment and a burden to the body. In fevers, the temperature goes up after feeding. This shows that more poison has entered the blood. In fevers little or none of the digestive fluids is secreted, but the alimentary tract is so warm that the food decomposes quickly. Feeding during acute attacks of disease is one of the most serious and fatal of errors. There is an aversion to food, which is nature's request that none be taken.

When an animal becomes seriously ill, it wants to fast, and does so unless man interferes. Here we could with advantage do as the animals do. Nature made no mistake when she took hunger away in acute diseases, and if we disregard her desires, we invariably suffer for it.

We should make it a rule to take no food, either liquid or solid, during acute disease.

Those who have had no opportunity to watch the rapidity with which people recover from serious illness may take the ground that sick people would starve to death if they were to be treated thus, for some of these acute diseases last a long time. Typhoid fever, for instance, occasionally lasts two or three months. It never lasts that long when treated by natural means, and it is very mild, as a rule. The fever will be gone in from seven to fourteen days in the vast majority of cases, and then feeding can be resumed.

Chronic disease is often due to neglected acute disease, at other times to the building of abnormality through errors of life which have not resulted in acute troubles. While acquiring chronic disease, the individual may be fairly comfortable, but he is never up to par. Most chronic diseases can be cured quickly by taking a fast, but usually it is not necessary to take a complete fast. The desire for food is not generally absent and there is usually fair power to digest. One of the most satisfactory methods, if not the most satisfactory one, of treating chronic disease is to reduce the food intake, and instead of giving so much of the concentrated staples, feed more of the succulent vegetables and the fresh fruits, cooked and raw, using but small quantities of flesh, bread, potatoes and sugar. This gives the body a chance to throw off impurities. There are always many impurities in a deranged body.

Third, Be moderate in your eating: This is often very difficult, for most people do not know what moderation is. In infancy the too frequent feeding and the overfeeding begin. The common belief that infants must be fed every two hours, or oftener, is acted upon. The result is that the child soon loses its normal hunger, which is replaced by abnormal hunger. When food is long withheld it begins to fret. The mother again feeds and there is peace for an hour or so. When mothers learn to feed their children three times a day and no more there will be a great decrease in infant ills and a falling off in the infant mortality. The healthiest children I have seen are fed but three times a day. They become used to it and expect no more.

Another thing that makes it difficult to be moderate is impoverishing the food through refinement and poor cooking. These processes take away a great part of the mineral salts which are present in foods in organic form. These salts can not be replaced by table salt, for sodium chloride is but one of many salts that the body needs and an excess of table salt does not make up for a deficiency in the others.

Children fed on refined, impoverished foods are not satisfied with a reasonable amount. There is something lacking and this makes itself known in cravings, which demand more food than is needed to nourish. I have noticed many times that children are satisfied with less of whole wheat bread than of white bread, and that the brown unpolished rice satisfies them more quickly and completely than the polished rice. In other words, depriving the foods of their salts is one of the factors that leads to overeating.

Simplicity is a great aid to moderation. It is also necessary to exercise the conservative measure, self-control. Some writers suggest to eat all that is desired and then fast at various intervals to overcome the effects of overeating. In other words, they advise to eat enough to become diseased and then fast to cure the trouble. This is better than to continue the eating when the evil results of an excessive food intake make themselves known, but it does not bring the best results. Such people have their spells of sickness, which are unnecessary. If they stop eating as soon as the disease makes itself known, it does not last long. By exercising self-control sickness will be warded off. By using will power daily it grows stronger and those who force themselves to be moderate at first, are in time rewarded by having moderation become second nature.

People should always stop eating before they are full. Those who eat until they are uncomfortable are gluttons. They should be classed with drunkards and drug addicts.

If discomfort follows a meal it is a sign of overeating. It would be well to read this in connection with the chapter that treats of overeating.

Fourth, Thoroughly masticate all food: Horace Fletcher has written a very enthusiastic book on this subject. Enthusiasm is apt to lead one astray, and even if thorough mastication will not do all that Mr. Fletcher believed, it is very important, and we owe Mr. Fletcher thanks for calling our attention to the subject forcibly.

Thorough mastication partially checks overeating.

Our foods have to be finely divided and subdivided or they can not be thoroughly acted upon by the digestive juices. The stomach is well muscled and churns the food about, helping to comminute it, but it can not take the place of the teeth. All foods should be thoroughly masticated. While the mastication is going on the saliva becomes mixed with the food. In the saliva is the ptyalin, which begins to digest the starch. Starch that is well masticated is not so liable to ferment as that which gets scant attention in the mouth. Starches and nuts need the most thorough mastication. If thorough mastication were the rule, meat gluttons would be fewer, for when flesh is well chewed large quantities cause nausea.

Milk digests best when it is rolled around in the mouth long enough to be mixed with saliva. To treat milk as a drink is a mistake, for it is a very nourishing food.

All kinds of nuts must be well masticated. If they are not they can not be well digested, for the digestive organs are unable to break down big pieces of the hard nut meats.

The succulent vegetables contain considerable starch. If mastication is slighted they often ferment enough to produce considerable gas.

Fruits are generally eaten too rapidly, and therefore often produce bad results. Even green fruits can be eaten with impunity if they are very thoroughly masticated.

Those who are fond enough of liquors to take an excess should sip their alcoholic beverages very slowly, tasting every drop before swallowing. This would decrease their consumption of liquor greatly.

Even water should not be gulped down. It should be taken rather slowly, especially on hot days. During hot weather many drink too much water. This tendency can usually be overcome by avoiding iced water and by drinking slowly.

These four rules should be a part of your vital knowledge. If you forget everything else in this book, please remember them and try to put them into practice:

Eat only when hungry. During acute illness fast. Be moderate in your eating. Thoroughly masticate all food.

CHAPTER IX.

CLASSIFICATION OF FOODS.

Food is anything which, when taken into the body under proper conditions, is broken down and taken into the blood and utilized for building, repairing or the production of heat or energy.

There are various forms of foods, which can be divided into two classes: First, nitrogenous foods or proteins. Second, carbonaceous, foods, under which caption come the sugars, starches and fats. Salts and water are not usually classified as foods, though they should be, for life is impossible without either.

The chief proteins are: First, the albuminoids, which are represented by the albumin in eggs, the casein in milk and cheese, the myosin of muscle and the gluten of wheat. Second, the gelatinoids, which are represented by the ossein of bones, which can be made into glue, and the collogen of tendons. Third, nitrogen extractives, which are the chief ingredients in beef tea. They are easily removed from flesh by soaking it while raw in cold water. They are rich in flavor and are stimulating. They have absolutely no food value. Beef tea, and other related extracts, are not foods. They are stimulants. In truth they are of no value, and those who purchase such preparations pay a high price and get nothing in return.

The sugars and starches are grouped under the name of carbohydrates, which means that they are a combination of water and carbon. There are various forms of sugar. About 4 per cent of milk is milk sugar, which agrees better with the young than any other kind of sugar. It is not so soluble in water as the refined cane sugar, and therefore not so sweet, but it is fully as nourishing. Honey is a mixture of various kinds of sugars. Cane sugar is taken principally from sugar beets and sugar cane. There is no chemical difference between the products of canes and beets. Sugars can not be utilized by the blood until it has changed them into other forms of sugar.

The use of sugar is rapidly increasing. Several centuries ago it was used as a drug. It was doubtless as effective as a curing agent as our drugs are today. Until within the last sixty or seventy years it has not been used as a staple food. Now it is one of our chief foods. Not so very long ago but ten pounds of sugar per capita were used annually, but now we are consuming about ninety pounds each annually, that is, about four ounces per day. Many people look upon sugar as a flavoring, which it is in a measure, but it is also one of our most concentrated foods.

That this great consumption of sugar is harmful there is no doubt. Physicians who practiced when the use of sugar was increasing very rapidly called attention to the increasing decay of teeth. Sugar, as it appears upon the table is an unsatisfied compound. It does not appear in concentrated form in nature, but mixed with vegetable and mineral matters, and when the pure sugar is put into solution it seeks these matters. It is especially hungry for calcium and will therefore rob the bones, the teeth and the blood of this important salt, if it can not be had otherwise. The most noticeable effect is the decay of the teeth.

I have read considerable literature of late blaming sugar for producing many diseases, among them tuberculosis and cancer. Improper feeding is the chief cause of these diseases, but to blame sugar for all ills of that kind is far from arriving at the truth. Cancer and tuberculosis killed vast numbers of people before sugar was used as a staple. If we wish to get at the root of any trouble, it is necessary for us to bury our prejudices and be broad minded.

People who eat much sugar should also partake liberally of fresh raw fruits and vegetables, in order to supply the salts in which sugar is deficient. Lump sugar is practically pure, and therefore a poorer article of diet than any other form of sugar, for man can not live on carbon without salts.

Grape sugar and fruit sugar are the same chemically. Another name for them is dextrose, and in the form of dextrose sugar is ready to be taken up by the blood.

Children like sweets, but it is just as easy to give them the sweet fruits, such as good figs, dates and raisins, as it is to give them commercial sugar and candy, and it is much better for their health. Children who get used to the sweet fruits do not care very much for candies. The sugar in these fruits is not concentrated enough to be an irritant and it contains the salts needed by the body. Hence it does not rob the body of any of its necessary constituents. Because the fruit sugar, taken in fruit form, is not so concentrated and irritating as the common sugar, the child is satisfied with less.

Sugar is an irritant of the mucous membrane and therefore stimulates the appetite. This is true only when it is taken in excess in its artificial form, and it does not matter whether it is sugar, jelly or jam. For this reason jellies and jams should be used sparingly, because it is not necessary to stimulate the appetite. Those who resort to stimulation overeat. When much sugar is taken, it not only irritates the stomach, but it even inflames this organ.

Sugar is a preservative, and like all other preservatives it delays digestion, if taken in great quantities, and four ounces per day make a great quantity. The digestive organs rebel if they are given as much of sugar as they will tolerate of starch. When taken in excess sugar ferments easily, producing much gas, which is followed by serious results.

Sugar is changed into forms less sweet by acids and heat. The ferment invertin also acts upon sugars.

Sugar is a valuable food, but we are abusing it, and therefore it is doing us physical harm. The quantity should be reduced, and families who are using four ounces per person per day, as statistics indicate that most are doing, should reduce the intake to about one-third of this amount. It would be well to take as much of the sugar as possible in the form of sweet fruits.

It is a fact that sugar is easy to digest and that one can soon get energy from it, but feeding is not merely a question of giving digestible aliments, but a question of using foods that are beneficial in the long run. The moderate use of this food is all right, but excess is always bad. Starches need more change than sugars before they can be absorbed by the blood, but they give better results. Chemically there is but small difference between starch and sugar. The starch must be changed into dextrose, a form of sugar, before it can be utilized by the body.

The human body contains a small amount of a substance called glycogen, which is an animal starch or sugar. This glycogen is burned. Sugar is a force food. It combines with oxygen and gives heat and energy. The waste product is carbonic acid gas, which is carried by the blood to the lungs and then exhaled.

Honey and maple sugar are good foods, but overconsumption is harmful.

Sugar eating is largely a habit. Because the sugar has so much of the life and so many of the necessary salts removed in its refinement it is a good food only when taken in small quantities. Nature demands of us that we do not get too refined in our habits, for excessive refinement is followed by decay. It is easy to overcome the tendency to overeat of sugar.

Some spoil the most delicious watermelon by heaping sugar or salt, or both, upon it. In this way the flavor is lost. There is not a raw fruit on the market which is as finely flavored after it has been sugared as it was before. True, those who have ruined their sense of taste object to the tartness and natural acidity of various foods, but they are not judges and can not be until they have regained a normal taste, which can only be done by living on natural foods for a while.

Fats are obtained most plentifully from nuts, legumes, dairy products and animal foods. They are the most concentrated of all foods, yielding over twice the amount of heat or energy that we can obtain from the same weight of pure sugar, starch or protein. Many who think they are moderate eaters consume enough butter to put them in the glutton class.

Salts are present in all natural foods of which we partake.

Water is indispensable, for the body has to have fluids in order to perform its functions.

Foods are burned in the body. They are valuable in proportion to the completeness with which they are digested and assimilated and the ease with which this process is accomplished. It takes energy to digest food and if the food is very indigestible it takes too much energy.

The following remarks on digestibility are according to the best knowledge we have on the subject:

As a general rule, the protein of meat and fish is more completely and more quickly digested than the protein in vegetable foods. The reason is that the vegetable protein is found in cells which are protected by the indigestible cellulose which covers each cell. This covering is not always broken and then the digestive juices are practically powerless.

The legumes, which are rich in protein, are comparatively hard to digest. If properly prepared and eaten, they give little or no trouble, but they are generally cooked soft and the mastication is slighted. The result is fermentation. Beans, peas and lentils should be very well chewed, and eaten in moderation, for they are rich both in starch and protein.

Nuts are as a rule not as completely digested as meats and animal fats, and the principal reason is that they are eaten too rapidly and masticated too little. Nuts properly masticated, taken in correct combinations and amounts agree very well. It is not necessary, as many believe, to salt them in order to prevent indigestion.

In the following pages will be found a number of diet tables, giving compositions and fuel values of various foods which have been grouped for the sake of convenience, for the foods in each group are quite similar. These tables are not complete, for to list every food would take too much space. I have simply selected a representative list from the various classes of foods. Under flesh are given fish, meats and eggs. Under succulent vegetables are given both root and top vegetables, because of their similarity. Nuts, cereals, legumes, tubers and fruits are each grouped because it is easy to gain an understanding of them in this way. Milk is given a rather long chapter of its own because of its great importance in the morning of life.

Allow me to repeat that it is impossible to figure out the calories in a given amount of food and then give enough food to furnish so many calories and thus obtain good results. I have already given the key to the amount of food to eat, and it is the only kind of key that works well. However, it is very helpful to have a knowledge of food values.

The calorie is the unit of heat, and heat is convertible into energy. A calorie is the heat required to raise the temperature of one kilogram of water one degree C. To translate into common terms, it is the heat required to raise one pound of water four degrees F.

One pound of protein produces 1,860 calories. One pound of sugar produces 1,860 calories. One pound of starch produces 1,860 calories. One pound of oil or fat produces 4,220 calories.

For the scientific facts regarding foods I have consulted various works, especially the following: Diet and Dietetics, by Gauthier; Foods, by Tibbles; Food Inspection and Analyses, by Leach; Foods and their Adulteration, by Wiley; Commercial Organic Analysis, by Allan. However, I am most indebted to the numerous bulletins issued by the U. S. Department of Agriculture. All who make a study of foods and their value owe a great debt to W. O. Atwater and Chas. D. Wood, who have worked so long and faithfully to increase our knowledge regarding foods.

As we consider the various groups of foods, directions are given for the best way of cooking, but no fancy cooking is considered. Those who wish fancy, indigestible dishes should consult the popular cook books.

The women have it in their power to raise the health standard fifty to one hundred per cent by cooking for health instead of catering to spoiled palates, and by learning to combine foods more sensibly than they have in the past. The art of cooking has made its appeal almost entirely to the palate. This art is not on as high level as the science of cooking, which gives foods that build healthy bodies. The right way of cooking is simpler, quicker and easier than the conventional method, and gives food that is superior in flavor. After the normal taste has been ruined, it takes a few months to acquire a natural taste again so that good foods will be enjoyed.

CHAPTER X.

FLESH FOODS.

===
===== Pro- Carbohy- Calories Water tein Fat drates Ash per lb. --------------------
--- Beef, average 72.03 21.42 5.41 .... 1.14 .... Veal, lean 78.84 19.86 .82 .... .50 .... Mutton, average 75.99 17.11 5.77 .... 1.33 .... Pork, average fat 47.40 14.54 37.34 .... .72 .... Pork, average lean 72.57 20.25 6.81 .... 1.10 .... Rabbit 66.80 22.22 9.76 .... 1.17 .... Chicken, fat 70.06 19.59 9.34 .... .91 .... Turkey 65.60 24.70 8.50 .... 1.20 .... Goose 38.02 15.91 45.59 .... .49 .... Pigeon 75.10 22.90 1.00 .... 1.00 .... Duck, wild 69.89 25.49 3.69 .... .93 .... Black bass 76.7 20.4 1.7 .... 1.2 450 Sea bass 79.3 18.8 .5 .... 1.4 370 Cod, steaks 82.5 16.3 .3 .... .9 315 Halibut, steaks 75.4 18.3 5.2 .... 1.1 560 Herring 74.67 14.55 9.03 .... 1.78 .... Mackerel 73.4 18.2 7.1 .... 1.3 640 Perch, white 75.7 19.1 4.0 .... 1.2 525 Pickerel 79.8 18.6 .5 .... 1.1 365 Salmon 71.4 19.9 7.4 .... 1.3 680 Salmon trout 69.1 18.2 11.4 .... 1.3 820 Shad 70.6 18.6 9.5 .... 1.3 745 Sturgeon 78.7 18.0 1.9 .... 1.4 415 Trout, brook 77.8 18.9 2.1 .... 1.2 440 Clams, long 85.8 8.6 1.0 2.00 2.6 240 Clams, round 86.2 6.5 .4 4.20 2.7 215 Lobster 79.2 16.4 1.8 .40 2.2 390 Oyster in shell 86.9 6.2 1.2 3.70 2.0 230 --

The food value of meat depends on the amount of fat and protein it contains. Lean meat may contain less than four hundred calories per pound, while very fat meat may contain more than one thousand five hundred calories.

These foods are eaten because they are rich in protein. Protein is the great builder and repairer of the body. It forms the framework for both bone and muscle. We can get along very well without starch or sugar or fat, but it is absolutely necessary to have proteid foods. They are the only ones that contain nitrogen, which is essential to animal life.

Nitrogenous foods are used not only to build and repair, but in the end they are burned, supplying as much heat as the same weight of sugar or starch.

Proteid foods are generally taken to excess. To most people they are very palatable, and they are generally prepared in a manner that renders rapid eating easy. Besides, meats contain flavoring and stimulating principles, called extractives, which increase the desire for them. The consequence is that those who eat meat often have a tendency to eat too much. Excessive meat eating often leads to consumption of large quantities of liquor. Stimulants crave company.

As will be noted, most fish and meat contain about 20 per cent. of protein, while about 75 per cent. is water. The fatter the meat, the less water it contains, and the more fuel value it has. The leaner the meat, the more watery the animal, and the more easily is the flesh digested. Beef is fatter than veal and harder to digest. Also, the flesh of old animals is more highly flavored than that of the young ones, because it contains more salts. For this reason people who have a tendency to the formation of foreign deposits, as is the case with those who have rheumatism and gout or hardening of the arteries, should take the flesh of young animals when it is obtainable.

In the past we have been taught to partake of excessive amounts of protein. The prescribed amount for the average adult has been about five ounces. If we were to obtain all the protein from meat, this would necessitate eating about twenty-five ounces of meat daily. However, inasmuch as there is considerable protein in the cereals and milk, and a little in most fruits and vegetables, a pound of meat would probably suffice under the old plan. A few physicians have known that such an intake of protein is excessive, and now the physiologists are learning the same. It has lately been determined experimentally that the body needs only about an ounce of protein daily, which will be supplied by about five ounces of flesh. Three or four ounces of flesh daily make a liberal allowance, for it is supplemented by protein in other foods.

Workers eat large quantities of flesh because they think they need a great deal. The fact is that very little more protein is needed by those who do hard physical labor than by brain workers. The extra energy needed calls for more carbohydrates, not for protein.

When the organism is supplied with sugar, starch and fat, or one of these, the protein of the body is saved, only a very small amount being used to replace the waste through wear and tear. Though protein can be burned in the body, it is not an economical fuel, either from a physiological or financial standpoint. The energy obtained from flesh costs much more than the same amount of energy obtained from carbonaceous foods. Ten acres of ground well cultivated can raise enough cereals and vegetables to support a number of people, but if this amount of land is used for raising animals, it will support but a few. The protein obtained from peas, beans and lentils is cheap, but these foods do not appeal to the popular palate as much as flesh.

Meat immediately after being killed is soft. After a while it goes into a state of rigidity known as rigor mortis. Then it begins to soften again. This third stage is really a form of decay, called ripening. It is believed that the lactic acid formed is one of the principal agents producing this softening. Some people enjoy their meats, especially that of fowls and game, ripe enough to deserve the name of rotten. The ripening produces many chemical changes in the meat, which give the flesh more flavor. Consequently those who indulge are very apt to overeat. It is a fact that those who eat much flesh go into degeneration more quickly than those who are moderate flesh eaters and depend largely on the vegetable kingdom for food.

If an excess of good meat causes degeneration, there is no reason to doubt that partaking of overripe foods is even worse.

All meat contains waste. If the flesh comes from healthy animals and is eaten in moderation this waste is so small that it will cause no inconvenience, for a healthy body is able to take care of it. If too much is eaten, the results are serious. Overeating of flesh is followed by excessive production of urea and uric acid products. Some of these may be deposited in various parts of the body, while the urea is mostly excreted by the kidneys. The kidneys do not thrive under overwork any more than other organs. The vast majority of cases of diabetes and Bright's disease are caused by overworking the digestive organs. Too much food is absorbed into the blood and the excretory organs have to work overtime to get rid of the excess.

Meats are easily spoiled. They should be kept in a cold place and not very long. Fresh meat and fish are more easily digested than those which are salted, or preserved in any other way. Pickled meats should be used rarely The same is true of fish.

Ptomaines, or animal poisons, form easily in flesh foods. These are very dangerous, and it is not safe to eat tainted flesh, even after it is cooked. Fish decomposes quickly and fish poisoning is probably even more severe than meat poisoning. Fish should be killed immediately after it is caught, for experiments have shown that the flesh of fish kept captive after the manner of fishers degenerates very rapidly. Fish should be eaten while fresh. Even when the best precautions have been taken, it is somewhat risky to partake of fish that has been shipped from afar.

Flesh foods are more easily and completely digested than the protein derived from the vegetable kingdom.

From the table it will be noted that some fish is fat and some is lean. The ones containing more than 5 per cent of fat should be considered fat fish. These are somewhat harder to digest than the lean ones, but they are more nutritious.

Shell fish is generally low in food value and if taken as nourishment is very expensive. However, most people eat this food for its flavor.

COOKING.

Cooking is an art that should be learned according to correct principles. Every physician should be a good cook. He should be able to go into the kitchen and show the housewife how to prepare foods properly. Medical men who are well versed in food preparation and able to make good food prescriptions have no need of drugs.

The flesh of animals is composed of fibres. These fibres are surrounded by connective tissue which is tough. The cooking softens and breaks down these tissues, thus rendering it easier for the digestive juices to penetrate and dissolve them. That is, proper cooking does this. Poor cooking generally renders the meats indigestible.

The simpler the cooking, the more digestible will be the food. Flavors are developed in the process, but these are hidden if the meats are highly seasoned.

Boiling: When meats are boiled they lose muscle sugar, flavoring extracts, organic acids, gelatin, mineral matters and soluble albumin. That is, they lose both flavor and nourishment. Therefore the liquid in which they are cooked should be used.

The proper way to boil meat is to plunge it into plain boiling water. Allow the water to boil hard for ten or fifteen minutes. This coagulates the outer part of the piece of meat. Then lower the temperature of the water to about 180 degrees F. and cook until it suits the taste. If it is allowed to boil at a high temperature a long time, it becomes tough, for the albumin will coagulate throughout.

Salt extracts the water from meat. Therefore none of it should be used in boiling. The meat should be cooked in plain water with no addition. No vegetables and no cereals are to be added. All meats contain some fat, and this comes into the water and acts upon the vegetables and starches, making them indigestible. Season the meat after it is cooked, or better still, let everyone season it to suit the taste after serving.

Meats that are to be boiled should never be soaked, for the cold water dissolves out some of the salts and some of the flavoring extracts, as well as a part of the nutritive substances. It is better to simply wash the meat if it does not look fresh and clean enough to appeal to the eye, which it always should be.

Stewing: If meat is to be stewed, cut into small pieces and stew or simmer at a temperature of about 180 degrees F. until it is tender. It is to be stewed in plain water. If a meat and vegetable stew is desired, stew the vegetables in one dish, and the meat in another. When both are done, mix. By cooking thus a stew is made that will not "repeat" if it is properly eaten. Foods should taste while being eaten, not afterwards.

Broths: If a broth is desired, select lean meat. Either grind it or chop it up fine. There is no objection to soaking the meat in cold water, provided this water is used in making the broth. Use no seasoning. Let it stew or simmer at about 180 degrees F. until the strength of the meat is largely in the water.

When the broth is done, set it aside to cool. Then skim off all the fat and warm it up and use. One pound of lean meat will produce a quart of quite strong broth.

Broiling: Cut the meat into desired thickness. Place near intense fire, turning occasionally, until done. Be careful not to burn the flesh. An ordinary steak should be broiled in about ten minutes. Of course, the time depends on the thickness of the cut and whether it is desired rare, medium or well done, and in this let the individual suit himself, for he will digest the meat best the way he enjoys it most.

Beefsteak smothered in onions is a favorite dish. It is not a good way to prepare either the onions or the steak. A better way is to broil both the steak and the onions, or broil the steak, cut the onions in slices about one-half to three-fourths of an inch thick, add a little water and bake them. Beefsteak and onions prepared in this way are both palatable and easy to digest.

Roasting is just like broiling, that is, cooking a piece of meat before an open fire. Here we use a larger piece of meat and it therefore takes longer. Of old roasting was quite common, but now we seldom roast meat in this country.

Baking: Here we place the meat in an enclosed oven. Most of our so-called roast meats are baked. The oven for the first ten or fifteen minutes should be very hot, about 400 degrees F. This heat seals the outside of the meat up quite well. Then let the heat be reduced to about 260 degrees F. If it is kept at a high temperature it will produce a tough piece of meat. The time the meat should be in the oven depends upon the size of the piece of meat and how well done it is desired.

While baking, some of the juices and a part of the fat escape. About every fifteen minutes, baste the meat with its own juice. A few minutes before the meat is to be removed from the oven it may be sprinkled with a small amount of salt, and so may broiled and roasted meats a little while before they are done. However, many prefer to season their own foods or eat them without seasoning and they should be allowed to do so.

Steaming: This is an excellent way of cooking. None of the food value is lost. Put the meat in the steamer and allow it to remain until done. The cheapest and toughest cuts of meat, which are fully as good as the more expensive ones and often better flavored, can be rendered very tender by steaming. Tough birds can be treated in the same way. An excellent way to cook an old hen or an old turkey is to steam until tender and then put into a hot oven for a few minutes to brown. Some birds are so tough that they can not be made eatable by either boiling or baking, but steaming makes them tender.

It is best to avoid starchy dressings, in fact dressings of all kinds. A well cooked bird needs none, and dressing does not save a poorly cooked one. Most dressings are very difficult to digest.

Fireless cooking: Every household should have either a good steamer or a fireless cooker. Both are savers of time and fuel and food. They emancipate the women. Those who have fireless cookers and plan their meals properly do not need to spend much time in the kitchen.

Place the meat in the fireless cooker, following the directions which accompany it. However, if they tell you to season the meat, omit this part.

Smothering is a modification of baking. Any kind of meat may be smothered, but it is especially fine for chickens. Take a young bird, separate it into joints, place into a pan, add a pint of boiling water. If chicken is lean put in a little butter, but if fat use no butter. Cover the pan tightly and place in oven and let it bake. A chicken weighing two and one-half pounds when dressed will require baking for one hour and fifteen minutes. Keep the cover on the baking pan until the chicken is done, not raising it even once. Gravy will be found in the pan.

Pressed chicken is very good. Get a hen about a year old. Place it into steamer or fireless cooker until so tender that the flesh readily falls from the bones. Remove the bones, but keep the skin with the meat. Chop it up. Place in dish or jar, salting very lightly. Over the chopped-up meat place a plate and on this a weight, and allow it to press over night. Then it is ready to slice and serve. This is very convenient for outings.

Fish should preferably be baked or broiled. It may also be boiled, but it boils to pieces rather easily and loses a part of its food value. It must be handled with great care. No seasoning is to be used. When served a little salt and drawn butter or oil may be added as dressing.

Frying is an objectionable method of cooking. It is generally held, and with good reason, that when grease at a high temperature is forced into flesh, it becomes very indigestible. In fact the crust formed on the outside of the flesh can not be digested. It is folly to prepare food so that it proves injurious.

However, there is a way of using the frying pan so that practically no harm is done. Grease the pan very lightly, just enough to prevent the flesh from sticking. Make the pan very hot and place the meat in it. Turn the meat frequently. Fries (young chickens) may be cooked in this way with good results. The same is true of steaks and chops.

Avoid greasy cooking. It is an abomination that helps to kill thousands of people annually.

Paper bag cooking is all right if it is convenient. Those who have good steamers or fireless cookers will not find it of special advantage.

Brown flour gravies are not fit to eat. If there is any gravy serve it as it comes from the pan without mixing it with flour or other starches. It may be put over the meat or used as dressing for the vegetables. Milk gravies are also to be avoided. Use only the natural gravies.

Oysters may be eaten raw or stewed. Stew the oysters in a little water. Heat the milk and mix. Eat with cooked succulent vegetables and with raw salad vegetables. It is best to leave the crackers out. The oysters themselves contain very little nourishment, but when made into a milk stew the result is very nutritious.

Eggs should be fresh. Some bakers buy spoiled eggs and use them for their fancy cakes and cookies. This is a very objectionable practice and may be one of the reasons that bakers' cookies never taste like those "mother used to make." Eggs take the place of fish, meat or nuts, for they are rich in protein. They may be taken raw, rare or well done.

Eggs may be boiled, poached, steamed or baked. Soft boiled eggs require about three and one-half minutes. Hard boiled ones require from fifteen to twenty minutes. The albumin of an egg boiled six or seven minutes is tough. When boiled longer it becomes mellow. Eggs may be made into omelettes or scrambled, but the pan should be lightly greased and quite hot so that the cooking will be quickly done. Eggs are variously treated for an omelette. Some cooks add nothing but water and this makes a delicate dish. Others use milk, cream or butter, and beat.

Bacon is a relish and may be taken occasionally with any other food. It should be well done, fried or broiled until quite crisp. This is one place where frying is not objectionable.

Pork should rarely be used. It is too fat and rich and requires too long to digest. When eaten it should be taken in the simplest of combinations, such as pork and succulent vegetables or juicy fruits, either cooked or raw, and nothing else.

Flesh may be eaten more freely in winter than in summer. Meat especially should be eaten very sparingly during hot weather, for it is too stimulating and heating. Nuts, eggs and fish are then better forms in which to take protein.

COMBINATIONS.

Flesh foods combine best with the succulent vegetables and the salad vegetables or with juicy fruits. It is more usual to take vegetables with flesh than to take fruit, but those who prefer fruit may take it with equally as good results. Both fruits and vegetables are rich in tissue salts, in which flesh foods are rather deficient. The succulent vegetables contain some starch and the juicy fruits some sugar, but not enough to do any harm. They both act as fillers.

Flesh is quite concentrated and it is customary to take it with other concentrated foods, such as bread and potatoes. As a result too much food is ingested. It would be a splendid rule to make to avoid bread and potatoes when flesh food is taken, but if this seems too rigid, make it a rule never to eat all three at the same meal. It is best to eat the flesh foods without bread or potatoes, but if starch is desired, take only one kind at a time.

Most people crave a certain amount of food as filler, and they have fallen into the habit of using bread and potatoes for this purpose. This is a mistake. Use the juicy fruits and the succulent vegetables for filling purposes and thus get sufficient salts and avoid the many ills that come from eating great quantities of concentrated foods.

When possible, have a raw salad vegetable or two with the meat or fish meal.

Eat only one concentrated albuminous food at a meal. If you have meat, take no fish, eggs, nuts or cheese.

CHAPTER XI.

NUTS.

	Water	Protein	Fat	Carbohydrates	Ash	Calories per lb.
Acorns	4.1	8.1	37.4	48.0	2.4	2718
Almonds	4.8	21.0	54.9	17.3	2.0	3030
Brazil nuts	5.3	17.0	66.8	7.0	3.9	3329
Filberts	3.7	15.6	65.3	13.0	2.4	3432
Hickory nuts	3.7	15.4	67.4	11.4	2.1	3495
Pecans	3.0	11.0	71.2	13.3	1.5	3633
English walnuts	2.8	16.7	64.4	14.8	1.3	3305
Chestnuts, dried	5.9	10.7	7.0	74.2	2.2	1875
Butternuts	4.5	27.9	61.2	3.4	3.0	3371
Cocoanuts	14.1	5.7	50.6	27.9	1.7	2986
Pistachio nuts	4.2	22.6	54.5	15.6	3.1	3010
Peanuts, roasted	1.6	30.5	49.2	16.2	2.5	3177

Nuts vary a great deal in composition. They are generally the seeds of trees, enclosed in shells, but other substances are also called nuts. The representative nuts are rich in fat and protein, containing some carbohydrate (sugar or starch.)

A few nuts, such as the acorn, cocoanut and chestnut, are very rich in starch, and these should be classified as starchy foods. Very few foods contain as high per cent of starch as the dry chestnut. In southern Europe chestnuts are made into flour, and this is made into bread or cakes. An inferior bread is also made of acorn flour. Chestnuts may be boiled or roasted. They are very nutritious.

The more representative nuts are pecans, filberts, Brazil nuts and walnuts. These may be used in place of flesh foods, for they furnish both protein and fats. If the kernel is surrounded by a tough membrane, as is the case in walnuts and almonds, it should be blanched, which consists in putting the kernel in very hot water for a little while and then removing this membrane. The pecan, though it does not contain very much protein, is one of the best nuts, one which can be eaten often without producing dislike.

Nuts have the reputation of being hard to digest. If they are not well masticated they are very hard to digest indeed, but when they are well masticated they digest almost as completely as do flesh foods and they produce no digestive troubles.

One reason that nuts have obtained a bad reputation is that they are often eaten at the end of a heavy meal, when perhaps two or three times too much food has already been ingested. The result is indigestion and the sufferer swears off on nuts. If he had sense enough to reduce his intake of bread, potatoes, meat, pudding and coffee, the benefit would be very great. The tendency is for the sufferer from indigestion to pick out a certain food and blame all the trouble on that, when in truth the combinations and the quantity of food are to blame.

Some vegetarians make nuts one of their principal foods. We can easily get along without flesh, for we can obtain all the protein needed from milk, eggs, nuts and legumes. However, people who are used to flesh are able to digest it when they can take hardly anything else. The foods which we prefer are taken largely because we have become accustomed to them and have formed a liking for them, not because they are the very best from which to select.

COOKING.

Nut butter: Take the nut meats, clean away all the skins and grind fine in a nut mill. Then form into a pasty substance with or without the addition of oil or water, to suit the individual taste. Most nut butters are very agreeable in flavor. Sometimes the nuts are roasted and sometimes they are not. Almond butter is very good. The nut butters soon spoil if left exposed to the air, for the oils they contain turn rancid.

Peanut butter can be made by taking clean kernels of freshly roasted peanuts and grinding fine. Some are very fond of this butter. Cocoanut and cocoa butters are not made in this way. They are purified fats, the former from cocoanuts, the latter from the cocoa bean.

Nut milk: Take nut butter and mix with water until it is of the desired consistency. Cocoanuts contain a sweet liquid which is called cocoanut milk. However, the artificial cocoanut milk is made by pouring a pint of boiling water over the flesh of a freshly grated cocoanut. Let it stand until cold and strain. If it is allowed to stand some hours the fat will rise to the top and form cream. This milk is used by some who object to the use of animal products.

Various meals are made from nuts and made into food for the sick. This does no harm, nor does it do any special good. These meals contain more or less starch and the action of starches is much the same, no matter what the source. Please remember that there are no health foods.

COMBINATIONS.

Nuts are especially fine in combination with fruits. Fresh pecan meats and mild apples make a meal fit for the gods. Nuts may be used in any combination in which flesh is used, that is, they take the place of flesh foods. The starchy nuts take the place of starchy foods.

A good meal is made of a fruit salad, consisting of two or three kinds of fresh fruits and nuts.

Nuts or nut butter with toast also make a good meal.

Nuts have such fine flavor that cooks should think twice before spoiling them. It is very difficult to use them in cookery and get a product that is as finely flavored as the original nuts. The vegetarians use them in compounding what they call roasts, cutlets, steaks, etc. My experience with these imitation products has not been of the best, for though my digestive organs are strong, they do not take kindly to these mixtures. Some of my friends report the same results, in spite of thorough mastication and moderation. These imitation roasts and cutlets usually contain much starch and there is no reason to believe that it is better to cook nut oils into starchy foods than it is to use any other form of fat for this purpose. Those who like starch and nuts can make a splendid meal of nut meats and whole wheat biscuits or zwieback.

In eating nuts, always remember that the mastication must be thorough. It takes grinding to break up the solid nut meats and the stomach and bowels have no teeth. Those who can not chew well should use the nuts in the form of butter.

Ordinarily two ounces of nut meats, or less, are sufficient for a meal.

At present prices, nuts are not expensive, as compared with meat. Meat is mostly water. Lean meat produces from five to seven hundred calories to the pound. Nut meats produce from twenty-seven to thirty-three hundred calories per pound. In other words, a pound of nut meats has the same fuel value as about five pounds of lean meat, but not as great protein value.

Those who are not used to nuts have a tendency to overeat, but this is largely overcome as soon as people become accustomed to them.

CHAPTER XII.

LEGUMES.

```
================================================================
===== Pro- Carbohy- Calories Water tein Fat drates Ash per lb. --------------------
-------------------------------------------------- Fresh Legumes: String beans ......... 89.2
```

2.3 0.3 7.4 0.8 195 Shelled limas .... 68.5 7.1 0.7 22.0 1.7 570 Shelled peas 74.6 7.0 0.5 16.9 1.0 465

Dried Legumes:

Lima beans .... 10.4 18.1 1.5 65.9 4.1 1625 Navy beans .... 12.6 22.5 1.8 59.6 3.5 1605 Lentils .... 8.4 25.7 1.0 59.2 5.7 1620 Dried peas .... 9.5 24.6 1.0 62.0 2.9 1655 Soy beans .... 10.8 34.0 16.8 33.7 4.7 1970 Peanuts .... 9.2 25.8 38.6 24.4 2.0 2560 -- -------------------------

Analyses of all foods are approximate. The food value varies with the conditions under which the foods are grown and is not always even approximately the same.

The fresh young legumes may be classed with the succulent vegetables. The matured, dried legumes are to be classed both as starchy and proteid foods. They are very easily raised and consequently cheap. They are the cheapest source of protein that we have. Peas and beans are very important foods in Europe. In this country we consume enormous quantities of beans. In Mexico they use a great deal of frijoles, the poor people having this bean at nearly every meal. In China they make the soy beans into various dishes. The lentil is much used in Europe and is gaining favor here, as it should, for it is splendid food, with a flavor of its own. Peanuts, which are really not nuts, but leguminous plants growing their seeds under the ground, are used extensively as food for man and beast.

These foods are much alike in composition, the soy bean being exceptionally rich in protein.

These foods have the undeserved reputation of being indigestible and of producing flatulence. They are a little more difficult to digest than some other foods, but they cause no trouble if they are taken in simple combinations and in moderation, provided they have been properly prepared.

It is necessary to masticate these foods very well, and avoid overeating. They are generally so soft that they are swallowed without proper mouth preparation. The result is that too much is taken of these rich foods, after which there is indigestion accompanied by gas production.

One rather peculiar food belonging to the legumes is the locust bean or St. John's bread, which we can sometimes obtain at the candy stores. It grows near the Mediterranean and is used in places for cattle feed. It is so sweet that it is eaten as a confection. Its name is due to the fact that they say St. John lived on this bean and wild honey. If he did he must have had a sweet tooth. Others say that the saint really devoured grasshoppers. It is not easy to decide, but I prefer to believe that he was a vegetarian.

COOKING.

The fresh young legumes are to be considered in the same class as succulent vegetables, which are dealt with in the next chapter.

Ripe peas, beans and lentils may be cooked alike.

In cooking ripe legumes, try to get as soft water as possible. Hard water contains salts of lime and magnesia and these prevent the softening of the legumes.

Bean soup: Clean the beans and wash them. Let them soak over night. Cook them in the same water in which they have been soaked, until tender. They are to be cooked in plain water without any seasoning and with the addition of neither fats, starches nor other vegetables. When the beans are done, meat stock and other vegetables may be added, if desired. Pea soup is made in the same way.

The reason for not draining away the water in which the beans are soaked is that it takes up some of the valuable salts, the phosphates for instance. The addition of seasoning or fat while they are cooking makes the beans indigestible.

Baked beans: Clean and wash well. Soak them over night. Let them boil about three and one-half to four hours, using the water in which they were soaked. Then put them into the oven to bake. They are to be cooked plain and no fat or seasoning is to be added while they are baking. After they are done you may add some form of fatty dressing, such as bacon, which has been stewed in a separate dish, or you may dress them with butter and salt when they are served. Cooked this way they digest much more easily than when cooked in the ordinary way with tomatoes and grease. Some prefer to add either sugar or molasses to the beans when they are put into the oven. Avoid too much sweetening. Lentils may be baked in the same way.

Boiled beans: The same as bean soup, except that less water is used. Dressing may be the same as for baked beans. Lentils and peas may be treated in the same way.

Beans and corn may be cooked together.

COMBINATIONS.

The legumes are so very rich that they should be eaten in very simple combinations. It is best to take them with some of the raw salad vegetables and nothing else, or with the raw salad vegetables and one of the stewed succulent vegetables. The legumes contain all the protein and all the force food the body needs, so it is useless to add meat, bread and potatoes. Tomatoes and other acid foods should not be used in the same meal, yet beans and tomatoes or beans and catsup are very common combinations.

A plate of bean soup makes a good lunch. Bean soup or baked or boiled beans with succulent vegetables, raw and cooked, give all the nourishment needed in a dinner.

Pea and bean flours can be purchased on the market. These flours can not be made into dough, but they may be used for thickening. They contain more protein than ordinary flour.

Both peas and beans may be roasted, but they are rather difficult to masticate. Roasted peas have a fine flavor. Roasted peanuts are a nutritious food, and may be taken in place of peas or beans.

More legumes and less flesh foods will help to reduce the cost of living. Taken in moderation and well masticated, the legumes are excellent foods.

CHAPTER XIII.

SUCCULENT VEGETABLES.

	Water	Protein	Fat	Carbohydrates	Ash	Calories per lb.
Asparagus	93.96	1.83	2.55	2.55	.67	.....
Beet	87.5	1.6	.01	8.8	1.10	215
Cabbage	90.52	2.39	.37	3.85	1.40	.....
Carrot	88.2	1.1	.4	8.2	1.00	219
Cauliflower	90.82	1.62	.79	4.94	.81	.....
Cucumber	95.4	.8	.2	3.1	.5	80
Egg plant	92.93	1.15	.31	4.34	.5	.....
Pumpkin	93.39	.91	.12	3.93	.67	.....
Lettuce	94.17	1.2	.3	2.9	.9	90
Okra	87.41	1.99	.4	6.04	.74	.....
Onion	87.6	1.6	.3	9.9	.6	225
Parsnip	83.0	1.6	.5	13.5	1.4	300
Radish	91.8	1.3	.3	8.3	1.0	135
Squash	88.3	1.4	.5	9.0	.8	215
Tomato	94.3	.9	.4	3.9	.5	105
Spinach	90.6	2.50	.5	3.8	1.7	.....
Kohlrabi	87.1	2.6	.2	7.1	1.7	.....

Lima beans and shelled peas are generally included in this list, though the young lima beans contain about 20 per cent. starch.

Look at the cabbage analysis for kale and Brussels sprouts. They are much alike.

Most of the vegetables contain from one-half of one per cent. to two per cent. of indigestible fibre, which is not listed above.

This is but a partial list of the succulent vegetables. In addition may be mentioned artichokes of the green or cone variety, chard, string beans, celery, corn on the cob, turnips, turnip tops, lotus, endive, dandelion and garlic.

These vegetables produce but little energy, for most of them are not rich in protein, fat and carbohydrates, but they have considerable salts, which are given in the tables as ash. Their juices help to keep the blood alkaline, and it would be well for people to get into the habit of eating these foods, not only cooked, but some of them raw. The salts are very easily disturbed and in cooking they are somewhat changed. The best salts we get when we consume natural foods, such as raw fruits and raw vegetables and milk.

Another function of the succulent vegetables is to take up space in the stomach. Many like to eat until they feel comfortably full, but if they indulge in concentrated foods to this extent they overeat. The succulent vegetables have the merit of taking up much space without furnishing very much nourishment and they should, therefore, be used as space-fillers. However, they contain enough nourishment to be well worth eating, and most of them are excellent in flavor. This flavor is not appreciated by those who eat much meat and drink much alcohol.

The liberal use of these cooked vegetables has a tendency to prevent constipation, and some of them are called laxative foods, such as stewed onions and spinach.

PREPARATION.

These vegetables may be either steamed or prepared in a fireless cooker.

The usual way is to cook them in water. Clean the vegetables. Then put them on to cook in enough water to keep from burning, but use no seasoning. When the vegetables are tender there should be only a little fluid left and those who eat of the vegetables should take their share of this fluid, for it may contain as high as one-half to two-thirds of the salts. When served, let each one season to taste. Avoid the use of vinegar and all other products of fermentation as much as possible. Lemon juice will furnish all the acid needed for dressing.

The vegetables may be dressed with salt, or salt and butter, or salt and olive oil, and at times with cream, or with the natural gravy from meats, but avoid the use of flour and milk dressings, usually called cream gravy. These vegetables may also be eaten without any dressing.

The water is drained off from corn on the cob, asparagus, artichokes and unpeeled beets.

Vegetables should not be soaked in water, for they lose a part of their value if this is done. Cucumbers may be soaked in water to remove a part of the rank flavor, before being peeled.

Spinach is prepared as follows: Wash thoroughly. Put about two tablespoonfuls of water in the bottom of the kettle. Put over the fire and let the spinach wilt. Its juice will then begin to pour out and the spinach will cook in its own juice. Let it cook slowly until tender. Serve the spinach with its proportion of the juice. At first this will taste rather strong, but after a while a person will not want the dry, tasteless mess that is drained, usually served in hotels and restaurants. If some of the roots are left on the spinach, it tastes milder. The roots contain sugar.

Some of these vegetables, such as summer squash, onions and parsnips may be baked. Onions are very good sliced and broiled, but they should never be fried. Beets are good baked, and especially is this true of sugar beets. Radishes are very delicate and delicious when peeled and boiled, but their preparation is tedious. Egg plant is to be stewed, but not fried. As usually served, dipped in egg, rolled in crumbs and fried it is very indigestible.

Beet greens are excellent. They are best if the beets are pulled very young and both the roots and the leaves are used. Turnip tops, dandelion, mustard and Swiss chard are other greens that are good. All of them are prepared like spinach, except that more water is necessary. However, do not use much water.

Those who say that the various vegetables are unfit to eat and act accordingly are missing some good food. The vegetables all contain crude fibre, but they hurt the stomach and intestinal walls no more than they hurt the mucous membrane of the tongue. They furnish some bulk for the intestines to act upon, which is good and proper. All animals need some bulky food, otherwise they become constipated.

Tomatoes are best raw. If they are stewed they are to be cooked plain. Adding crackers and bread crumbs is a mistake. They taste all right without sugar, but a little may be used as dressing.

Vegetable soup: Take equal parts of about four vegetables, any that you like. Slice and cook in plain water until tender. When done add enough water or hot milk to make it of the right consistency. Season to taste. One of the constituents may be starchy, such as potatoes, barley or rice, but the rest should be succulent vegetables.

COMBINATIONS.

The succulent vegetables may be combined with all other foods. They go well with flesh or milk or nuts or starchy foods. With flesh or nuts they make a very satisfying meal. They may be taken with fruit. The tomato grows as a vegetable, but for practical purposes it is a fruit. The tomato combines well with protein, but not so well with the starchy foods.

SALAD VEGETABLES.

If possible, salads should be made entirely of raw vegetables and raw fruits. The chief salad vegetables are celery, lettuce, tomatoes, cucumbers, cabbage, onions and garlic, the two last mentioned being used for flavoring.

Dr. Tilden, who has done much to popularize raw vegetable salads, has a favorite, which he calls by his own name. It is equal parts of lettuce, tomatoes and cucumbers, with a small piece of onion. Chop up coarse and dress with salt and olive oil and lemon juice. This is all right for those who like it, but many do not care for such a complex salad with such dressing. Some of the combination salads that are served are wonderful mixtures, containing as many as seven or eight vegetables and a complex dressing.

Raw onions are too irritating to use in large quantities, and the same is true of garlic. The best salads contain but two or three ingredients. Take any two of the vegetables mentioned, such as lettuce and tomatoes; lettuce and cucumbers; cabbage and celery; celery and tomatoes, or eat simply one of these green vegetables raw. It is a good thing to eat some of those salad vegetables daily. If your digestion is excellent, you may occasionally take raw carrots or turnips, and a few raw spinach leaves are tasty for a change. Never mind if people tease you about eating grass, for it helps you to keep well.

Dress the raw vegetables as your taste allows. Most people want some salt, or salt and lemon juice, or a little sugar, or cream, or salt and olive oil, or salt, olive oil and lemon juice, or mayonnaise on their salad vegetables. Some eat them without any dressing and the flavor is excellent. Tasty salad can be made of fruit and vegetables, using no dressing, but strewing some nuts over the dish. On warm days, such a salad makes a satisfactory lunch.

It is all right to make a fruit and vegetable salad. Instead of using tomatoes, take strawberries, apples, grapes, or any other acid fruit. These fruits may be combined with cabbage, lettuce, celery or cucumbers. Do not mix too many foods in a meal, for to do so is indicative of poor taste. Those with refined palates like simple meals, and there is no reason for making salads so complex, when simplicity is a requirement for building health. However, a complex salad made of raw vegetables and raw juicy fruits does not play so much havoc as a mixture of concentrated foods.

Lettuce and celery are the most satisfactory salad vegetables to mix with fruits.

People who eat raw fruits do not need to eat the raw salad vegetables, for fruits and vegetables supply the same salts. Those who avoid both raw fruits and raw vegetables are not treating their bodies fairly.

The vegetable salads are most satisfactory when taken in combination with flesh, nuts or eggs, together with cooked succulent vegetables. They may be eaten with starchy foods, but then they should contain little or no acid.

CHAPTER XIV.

CEREAL FOODS.

	Water	Protein	Fat	Carbohydrates	Ash
Barley.	10.9	12.4	1.8	72.5	2.4
Buckwheat.	12.6	10.0	2.2	73.2	2.0
Corn.	9.3	9.9	2.8	76.3	1.5
Kafir corn.	16.8	6.6	3.8	70.6	2.2
Oats.	11.0	11.8	5.0	69.2	3.0
Rice.	12.4	7.4	.4	79.4	.4
Rye.	11.6	10.6	1.0	73.7	1.9
Wheat, spring.	10.4	12.5	2.2	73.0	1.9
Wheat, winter.	10.5	11.8	2.1	73.8	1.8
First patent flour.	10.55	11.08	1.15	76.85	0.37
Whole wheat flour.	10.81	12.26	2.24	73.67	1.02
Graham flour.	8.61	12.65	2.44	74.58	1.72
Bread, ordinary white.	37.65	10.13	.64	51.14	.44
Bread, whole wheat.	41.31	10.60	1.04	46.11	.94
Bread, Graham.	42.20	10.65	1.12	44.58	1.45

The cereal foods are important because of their wide distribution and the ease with which they can be prepared and utilized as food. They are very productive and need but little care and hence are a cheap food. The body can digest and absorb sugar and starch more completely than any other kind of food.

All civilized people have a favorite cereal. The Chinese and Japanese use rice very extensively, and this grain is growing in favor with us. White people generally prefer wheat, which is an excellent grain that has been used by man for thousands of years. It has been found in ancient Egyptian tombs, and it is so retentive of life that it has started to grow after lying dormant for several thousand years. Truly it is a worthy food for man.

The table of cereals should be carefully studied. It will be seen that the grains contain much starch, a little fat, and considerable protein. They also carry sufficient of salts, but only a small amount of water.

Please note further that patent flour loses nearly all of its salts. Patent flour is the product that is left after all the bran and practically all of the germ have been removed from the wheat. Whole wheat flour, or entire wheat flour, is the name given to the flour that has had a great part of the outer covering of the wheat kernel removed. It is a misnomer. Graham flour, named after Dr. Graham, is the product of the whole wheat kernel, and it will be noted that it is richer in salts and protein than the white flour and the whole wheat flour. The whole wheat flour and Graham flour we find on the market are often the result of blending, which is also true of the patent flour.

As we would expect, the various breads are rich or poor in salts according to the flours from which they are made.

All the cereals are good foods, but inasmuch as wheat and rice are used most extensively, they will receive more attention than the rest.

Wheat is perhaps the best and most balanced of all our cereals. The whole wheat with the addition of a little milk is sufficient to support life indefinitely. It is one of the foods of which people never seem to tire. Tiring of food is often an indication of excess. It is with food as with amusement, if we get too much we become blase. Those who eat in moderation are content with simple foods, but those who eat too much want a great variety, as a rule. There are beef gluttons, who are satisfied with their flesh and liquor, but this is because the meats are so stimulating.

Inasmuch as we use so much wheat, it is important that we use it properly. Today people want refined foods, and in refining they spoil many of our best food products. Sugar is too refined for health, rice suffers through refinement, and so does wheat. The wheat kernel contains all the elements needed to support life. In making fine white flour of it, at least three-fourths of the essential salts are removed. This robs the wheat of a large part of its life-imparting elements, and makes of it starvation food. If much white bread is consumed it is necessary to supplement it by taking large quantities of fresh fruits and vegetables, not necessarily in the same meal, in order to get the salts that have been removed in the process of milling.

The salts are found principally in the coats of the wheat, and in removing these coats and the germ, not only the salts, but considerable protein is lost. In other words, we remove most of the essential salts and a considerable part of the building material of the wheat, and then we eat the inferior product. The finer and whiter the flour, the poorer it is.

White flour has a very high starch content. The products made from it are quite tasteless and lacking in flavor, unless flavoring is added. Those who are used to whole wheat products find the white bread flat. It is possible to consume large quantities of white bread, and yet not be satisfied. There is something lacking. Whole wheat bread is more satisfying and therefore the danger of overeating of it is not so great.

The advocates of white flour say that the bran is too irritating for the bowels and for this reason it should be rejected. There is no danger in eating the entire kernel, after it is ground up. The particles of bran are so fine that they do no harm. The intestines were evidently intended for a little roughage, and it might as well come partly from wheat as from other sources. The gentle stimulation produced by the bran helps to keep the intestines active. It is noticeable that consumption of very refined foods leads to constipation.

Bran bread and bran biscuits are prescribed for constipation. This is just as bad as removing the bran entirely. Man has never been able to improve on the composition of the wheat berry. When an excess of bran is eaten, it causes too great irritation and in the end the individual is worse off than before. The after effect of irritation is always depression and sluggishness. Recent experiments seem to show that it is not the coarseness of the bran that causes activity of the bowels, but that some of the contained salts are laxative, for the same results have been obtained by soaking the bran in water and drinking the liquid.

The products of refined flour are more completely and easily digested than the whole wheat products. However, by eating in moderation and masticating well every normal person is able to take good care of whole wheat products, and the benefit of using the entire grain is so great that we should hesitate about continuing the use of the refined flours and white breads.

In the French army it has been found that when the soldiers are fed on refined flour products they are not so well nourished as when they have whole wheat products, and that they must have more of other foods to supplement the impoverished breadstuffs. It is difficult to get people to realize how important it is to give the tissue salts with the foods. Salts are absolutely essential to vital activity, and a lack of salts always results in mental and physical depression and even in disease.

No matter what adults are given, children should not be fed on white flour products. They need all the salts in the wheat. Depriving them of salts retards their development and results in decaying teeth and poor bone formation, among other things. They do not feel satisfied with their white flour foods. Therefore they overeat and get indigestion, catarrh, adenoids and various other ills. It is not difficult for people with observing eyes to note the difference in satisfaction of children after they get impoverished foods and the natural foods.

Anemia is very common among children, especially among the girls. The chief reason is impoverished foods. Salts can be used by the animal organism only after they have been elaborated by the vegetable kingdom. To remove all the iron from wheat and then give inorganic iron, which can not be assimilated, in its stead, is the height of folly. By all means, use less of the white flour and more of the entire wheat flour. If the white flour habit can not be given up, take enough raw fruit and vegetables to make up for the loss of salts in milling.

When rice is properly prepared it digests very easily. It is a little poor in protein, but this can be remedied by taking some milk in the same meal.

The rice we ordinarily get is inferior to the natural product. First they remove the bran. Then the flour is taken off. Then it is coated with a mixture of glucose and talcum and polished. All this trouble is taken to make it appeal to the eye. This impoverished rice is lacking in salts. It will not support people in health. In the countries where polished rice is fed in great quantities, they suffer a great deal from degenerative diseases. One of these is beri-beri, in which there are muscular weakness and degeneration, indigestion, disturbances of the heart and often times anasarca. When people suffering from this disease are given those parts of the rice grain lost in making polished rice, they recover. This is proof enough that the cause of the disease is the impoverished food.

The rice that should be used is brown and unpolished. When it is cooked it looks quite white. It is very satisfying.

Rye is extensively used in some lands. The bread is very good. Oats are largely devoured in Scotland. Corn bread is a favorite food in the southern part of our country. The negroes are fond of corn and pork with molasses, which is far from an ideal combination in warm climates.

PREPARATIONS.

Wheat makes the best bread because it contains gluten. Among proteins gluten is unique, because it is so elastic and after it has stretched it has a tendency to retain its place. This is what makes bread so porous. There are various meals or flours that can not be made into bread, or even dough, because they lack compounds which will act as frame work.

Bread can be made in many ways. The chief question for the housewife to decide is whether to make the bread from entire wheat flour or from patent flour. They are so different in value that a decision should not be difficult. It is also necessary to decide whether to use yeast bread or some other kind.

Yeast bread is made essentially from flour, water and yeast in the presence of heat. There are so many ways of making bread of this kind that a recipe is not necessary. The amount of salt to be added depends upon individual taste. Some like to set their yeast working in part potato, part flour. Others use milk instead of water. Some add shortening. And nearly all women believe that their own bread is the best.

Yeast is made up of myriads of little plants or fungi, which thrive on the sugary part of the flour. They convert this into alcohol and carbonic acid gas. The alcohol is practically all gone before the bread is brought to the table. The gas raises the bread, assisted by the expansion of the water in the dough when it is placed in a hot oven.

The yeast consumes a great deal of the nutritive part of the flour. This may amount to from 5 to 8 per cent. of the food value, and I have read that sometimes it is as high as 20 per cent. Liebig said that the fermentation destroyed enough food material daily in Germany to supply 400,000 people with bread. However, yeast bread is very agreeable to the taste and therefore is probably worth more than the unfermented product.

One objection to yeast bread is that all the yeast is not killed in baking, and the alcoholic fermentation may start again in the stomach. If the bread is turned into zwieback this is remedied. Fresh bread is not fit to eat, for it is very rarely properly masticated and if it is merely moistened and converted into a soggy mass in the mouth it is hard to digest.

Unleavened bread is made by making the flour into a paste, rolling out thin and baking well. Any kind of flour may be used. This is the passover bread of the Jews.

Dr. Graham's bread was made by mixing Graham flour with water, without any leavening, mixing the dough thoroughly, putting this aside several hours and baking.

Macaroni and spaghetti are made by mixing durum wheat flour with water, without any leavening. With the addition of eggs we get commercial noodles. The paste is moulded as desired.

All bread stuffs should be well baked.. The baking turns part of the starch into dextrine, which is easy to digest. Biscuits should be placed into a hot oven, but bread should be put into an oven moderately heated, otherwise the crust forms too quickly.

Whenever a light product is desired, whether it is bread, biscuit or cake, sift the flour over and over again to get it well impregnated with air. The more air it contains the more porous will be the finished product. Five or six siftings will suffice.

Unleavened breads of excellent flavor can be made by using either cream or butter as shortening, rolling the bread very thin, like crackers, and baking thoroughly.

Shredded wheat biscuits, puffed wheat and puffed rice, flaked wheat and flaked corn are some of the good foods we can purchase ready made. Most of them should be placed in a warm oven long enough to crisp. Masticate thoroughly and take them with either butter or milk, or both. It is best to take the milk either before or after eating the cereal. Sugar should not be added to these foods. Those who are not hungry enough to eat them without sugar should fast until normal hunger returns.

Baking powder bread is very good. The essentials are well sifted flour, liquid, good baking powder, quick mixing and a hot oven. The following recipe, recommended by Dr. Tilden, is good: To a quart of very best flour, which has been sifted two or three times, add a little salt and a heaping teaspoonful of baking powder. Sift again three times. Then add one or two tablespoonfuls of soft butter. Mix rapidly into a rather stiff dough with unskimmed milk. The dough should be rolled thin, and cut into small biscuits or strips. Put into a pan and bake in a hot oven until there is a crisp crust on bottom and top, which will take about twenty minutes. The more thoroughly and quickly the dough is mixed, the better the result.

These biscuits or bread sticks are good, always best when made rather thin, not to exceed an inch in thickness after being baked. When an attempt is made to bake in the form of a fairly thick loaf it is generally a failure. Use the proportions of white and whole wheat flours desired.

If more butter or some cream is added and it is rolled out thin, it serves very well for the bread part of shortcake.

Toast: Slice any kind of bread fairly thin, preferably stale bread. Place the slices into a moderately hot oven and let them remain there until they are crisp through and through. The scorched bread that is generally served as toast is no better than untoasted bread.

Whole wheat muffins: One cup whole wheat flour; one cup white flour; one-fourth cup sugar; one teaspoonful salt; one cup milk; one egg; two tablespoonfuls melted butter; four teaspoonfuls baking powder. Mix dry ingredients; add milk gradually, then eggs and melted butter. Put into gem pans and bake in hot oven for twenty-five minutes.

Ginger bread: One cup molasses; one and three-fourths teaspoons soda; one-half cup sour milk; two cups flour; one-half teaspoon salt; one-third cup butter; two eggs; two teaspoonfuls ginger. Put butter and molasses in sauce pan and heat until boiling point is reached. Remove from fire, add soda and beat vigorously. Then add milk, egg well beaten, and remaining ingredients mixed and sifted. Bake twenty-five minutes in buttered, shallow pan in moderate oven.

Custard: Three cups milk; three eggs; one-half cup sugar; one-half teaspoonful vanilla; pinch of salt. Beat eggs, add sugar and salt; then add scalded milk and vanilla; mix well. Pour into cups, place them in a pan of hot water in oven and bake twenty to twenty-five minutes. Serve cold.

Custard may also be cooked in double boiler or baked in a large pan.

This is not a cereal dish, but the next one is.

Rice custard: To well cooked rice add a few raisins and a small amount of sugar. The raisins can be cooked with the rice or separately. Place the rice and raisins in a baking dish, pour over an equal amount of raw custard and bake as directed for custard. Bake in either individual cups or pan. When done the layer of custard is on top and the rice and raisins on the bottom.

Macaroni and cheese: Three-fourths cup macaroni broken in pieces; two quarts boiling water; one-half table-spoonful salt. Cook macaroni in salted water twenty minutes, or longer if necessary to make it tender; drain. Put layer of macaroni in buttered baking dish; sprinkle with cheese, and repeat, making the last or top layer of cheese. Pour in milk to almost cover. Put into oven and bake until the top layer of cheese is brown.

Corn bread: Two cups corn meal; one-half cup wheat flour; one tablespoonful sugar; one-half teaspoonful salt; two teaspoonfuls baking powder; two eggs; one and three-fourths cups milk. Sift corn meal, flour, baking powder, salt and sugar together four or five times; add eggs and milk; stir well, pour into a hot buttered pan; smooth the top with a little melted butter to crisp the crust. Bake a good brown in hot oven.

Another recipe for corn bread is: To one cup of wheat flour, add two cups of corn flour; two eggs; one heaping teaspoonful butter or cottolene; one heaping teaspoonful baking powder; one pinch soda, a scant fourth teaspoonful; one-half teaspoonful salt. Prepare and make into batter with milk and bake as directed in first recipe.

Corn mush: Cook corn meal in plain water until it is done. It may be cooked over the fire, in a fireless cooker or in a double boiler. Serve with rich milk; add a little salt if desired.

Oatmeal: Put into a double boiler and let it cook until it is very tender. It can also be cooked in a fireless cooker over night. It requires several hours cooking before it is fit to eat. All foods of this nature should be thoroughly cooked, and they may all be made into porridge, which is better.

The objection to all mushy foods is that they are hardly ever properly masticated. The result is that they ferment in the alimentary tract, especially when they are eaten with sugar, as they generally are. It is best to take the mushy foods with milk and a little salt or with butter. Eaten in this way there is not such tendency to overeat as when sugar is used. Children especially eat more of these foods than is good for them if they are allowed to take them with sweets. Porridge is more diluted than the mushes and hence the danger of overeating is not so great.

Boiled rice: The best way to cook it is in a double boiler or a fireless cooker. Every grain should be tender. Cook it in plan water. It is not necessary to stir, but if the rice becomes dry add some more water. If rice and milk are desired, warm the milk and add when the rice is done. Serve like oatmeal. Putting sugar on cereals is nonsense. They are very rich in starch and sugar is about the same as starch. Sugar stimulates the appetite, and consequently people who use it on cereals overeat of this concentrated food.

Rice and raisins: This is prepared the same as boiled rice, except that raisins are added to the rice and water when first put on to cook. With milk this makes a good breakfast or lunch.

COMBINATIONS.

Starches of the cereal order may be eaten in combination with fats, such as cream, butter, olive oil and other vegetable oils.

They combine well with all the dairy products, such as milk and cheese.

Starches combine well with nuts. Take a piece of whole wheat zwieback and some pecans, chew both the bread and the nuts well and you will find this an excellent meal.

There is nothing incompatible about eating cereals with flesh, but it generally leads to trouble, for people eat enough meat for a meal, and then they eat enough starch for a full meal. This overeating is injurious. Besides, starch digestion and meat digestion are different and carried on in different parts of the alimentary tract, so it is best to eat starchy foods and meats at different meals. Those who eat in moderation may eat starch and flesh in the same meal without getting into trouble.

In winter it is all right to take starch with the sweet fruits.

It is best to avoid mixing acid fruits and cereals. Even healthy people find that a breakfast of oranges and bread does not agree as well as one of milk and bread. The saliva, which contains ptyalin, is secreted in the mouth. The ptyalin starts starch digestion, but it does not work in the presence of acid. Eating acid fruits makes the mouth acid temporarily, and consequently the starch does not receive the benefit it should from mouth digestion. The result is an increased liability to fermentation in the alimentary tract.

To get the best results it is absolutely necessary to masticate all starchy foods well. If this is not done it is merely a question of time until there is indigestion, generally accompanied by much acidity and gas production. This condition is a builder of many ills.

Recipes for pies and cakes are not given in this book. The less these compounds are used the better. They are very popular and can be made according to directions in conventional cook books. Pies should be made with thin crusts, which should be baked crisp both on bottom and top. The best cakes are the plain ones.

When desserts are eaten, less should be taken of other foods. Most people make the mistake of eating more than enough of staple foods and then they add insult to injury by partaking of dessert.

CHAPTER XV.

TUBERS.

	Pro-tein	Fat	Carbohy-drates	Ash	Water	Calories per lb.
Potato............	2.2	0.1	18.0	1.0	78.3	375
Sweet potato......	3.0	2.1	42.1	.9	51.9	925
Jerusalem artichoke.	2.5	0.2	17.5	1.1	78.7	

The two tubers that are of chief interest are the Irish potato and the sweet potato. The former is easily and cheaply grown on vast areas of land and therefore forms a large part of the food of many people. Properly prepared it is easily digested and very nourishing.

The sweet potato is a richer food than the Irish potato, but on account of its high sugar contents people soon weary of it. The southern negroes are very fond of this food.

Like all other starches, potatoes must be thoroughly masticated, or they will disagree in time. Potatoes are of such consistency that they are easily bolted without proper mouth preparation. In time the digestive organs object.

A new tuber is receiving considerable attention. It is the dasheen. It is said to be of very agreeable flavor, mealy after cooking, and produces tops that can be used in the same manner as asparagus. The dasheen requires a rather warm climate for its growth.

PREPARATION.

Baking: All the tubers may be baked. Clean and place in the oven; bake until tender. A medium sized potato will bake in about an hour. If the potatoes are soggy after being baked they are not well flavored. To remedy this, run a fork into them after they have been in the oven for a while; this allows some of the steam to escape and the potatoes become mealy. When a fork can easily be run into the potato, it is well enough done.

If the potatoes are well cleaned, there is no objection to eating a part of the jacket after they are baked. The finest flavoring is right under the jacket. This part contains a large portion of the salts.

Boiling: All tubers may be boiled. It is best to keep the jacket on, otherwise a great deal of both the salts and the nourishment is lost. If the potatoes boiled in the jacket seem too highly flavored, cut off one of the ends before placing them in the water. It takes about thirty or forty minutes to boil a medium sized Irish potato. Test with a fork, the same as baked potato, to find if done.

Potatoes should never be peeled and soaked. If they are to be boiled without the jacket, they should be cooked immediately after being peeled.

Steamed potatoes are good.

There is no objection to mashing potatoes and adding milk, cream or butter, provided they are thoroughly masticated when eaten. If the potatoes are mashed, this should be so thoroughly done that not a lump is to be found.

Potatoes cooked in grease are an abomination. The grease ruins a part of the potato and makes the rest more difficult to digest. Potato chips, French fried potatoes and German fried potatoes are too hard to digest for people who live mostly indoors. They should be used very seldom.

COMBINATIONS.

Potatoes are best eaten in combinations such as given for cereals. They are commonly taken with meat and bread. This combination is one of the causes of overeating. Occasionally they may be eaten with flesh, but this should not be a habit. Take them as the main part of the meal. Baked potatoes and butter with a glass of milk make a very satisfying meal. A good dinner can be made of potatoes with cooked succulent vegetables and one or two of the raw salad vegetables, with the usual dressings. It is best not to eat potatoes and acid fruits in the same meal.

In selecting food it is well to remember that as a general rule but one heavy, concentrated food should be eaten at a meal, for when two, three or even four concentrated foods are partaken of, the appetite is so tempted and stimulated by each new dish that before one is aware of it an excessive amount of food has been ingested.

CHAPTER XVI.

FRUITS.

	Water	Protein	Etherial Extracts	Carbohy-drates	Ash	Calories per lb.
Apples	84.6	0.4	0.5	14.2	0.3	290
Bananas	75.3	1.3	0.6	22.0	0.8	460
Figs, fresh	79.1	1.5	...	18.8	0.6	380
Lemons	89.3	1.0	0.7	8.5	0.5	205
Muskmelons	89.5	0.6	...	9.3	0.6	185
Oranges	86.9	0.8	0.2	11.6	0.5	240
Peaches	89.4	0.7	0.1	9.4	0.4	190
Pears	80.9	1.0	0.5	17.2	0.4	...
Persimmons	66.1	0.8	0.7	31.5	0.9	630
Rhubarb, stalk	94.4	0.6	0.7	3.6	0.7	105
Strawberries	90.4	1.0	0.6	7.4	0.6	180
Watermelon	92.4	0.4	0.2	6.7	0.3	140

Dried Fruits:

Apples........... 26.1 1.6 2.2 68.1 2.0 1350 Apricots......... 29.4 4.7 1.0 62.5 2.4 1290 Citrons.......... 19.0 0.5 1.5 78.1 0.9 1525 Dates............ 15.4 2.1 2.8 78.4 1.3 1615 Figs............. 18.8 4.3 0.3 74.2 2.4 1475 Prunes........... 22.3 2.1 ... 73.3 2.3 1400 Raisins.......... 14.6 2.6 3.3 76.1 3.4 1605 Currants......... 17.2 2.4 1.7 74.2 4.5 1495 ---

Apricots, avocados, blackberries, cherries, cranberries, currants, gooseberries, grapes, huckleberries, mulberries, nectarines, olives, pineapples, plums, raspberries and whortleberries are some of the other juicy fruits. They are much like the apple in composition, containing much water and generally from 6 to 15 per cent of carbohydrates (sugar). Olives and avocados are rich in oil.

You may classify rhubarb, watermelons and muskmelons as vegetables, if you wish. On the table they seem more like fruit, which is the reason they are given here. Melons are fine hot weather food. They are mostly water, which is pure. During hot weather it is all right to make a meal of melons and nothing else, at any time. The melons are so watery that they dilute the gastric juice very much. The result is that when eaten with concentrated foods they are liable to repeat, which indicates indigestion.

Fruits are not generally eaten for the great amount of nourishment to be obtained from them. They are very pleasant in flavor and contain salts and acids which are needed by the body.

The various fluids of the body are alkaline, and the fruits furnish the salts that help to keep them so. A few secretions and excretions are naturally acid. Sometimes the body gets into a too acid state, but that is very rarely due to overeating of fruit. It is generally caused by pathological fermentation of food in the alimentary tract. The salts and acids of fruits are broken up in the stomach and help to form alkaline substances.

The water of the fruit is very pure, distilled by nature. The acid fruits are refreshing and helpful to those who have a tendency to be bilious. Fruits are cleansers, both of the alimentary tract and of the blood.

Fruits grow most abundantly in warm climates and that is where they should be used most. In temperate climates they should be eaten most freely during warm weather.

Young, vigorous people can eat all the fruit they wish at all seasons, within reason. Thin, nervous people, and those who are well advanced in years should do most of their fruit eating in summer. In winter there is a tendency to be chilly after a meal of acid fruit. In summer such meals do not add to the burden of life by making the partaker unduly warm.

The apple is perhaps the best all-round fruit of all. It is grown in many lands and climates. It is possible to get apples of various kinds, from those that are very tart to those that are so mild that the acid is hardly perceptible to the taste. Stout people can eat sour apples with benefit. Thin, fidgety ones should use the milder varieties. The juice from apples, sweet cider, freshly expressed, is a very pleasant drink, and may be taken with fruit meals.

The avocado is a good salad fruit. It is quite oily. A combination of avocado and lettuce makes a good salad.

Thanks to rapid transportation, the banana has become a staple. It is quite commonly believed that bananas are very starchy and rather indigestible. This may be true when they are green, but not when they are ripe. Green bananas are no more fit for food than are green apples. Ripe bananas are neither starchy nor indigestible. When the banana is ripe it contains a trace of starch, all the rest having been changed to sugar. A ripe banana is mellow and sweet, but firm. The skin is either entirely black, or black in spots, but the flesh is unspotted. The best bananas can often be purchased for one-half of the price of those that are not yet fit to eat.

Bananas are a rich food. Weight for weight they contain more nourishment than Irish potatoes. A few nuts or a glass of milk and bananas make a good meal. Bananas contain so much sugar that it is not necessary to eat bread or other starches with them. Those with normal taste will not spoil good bananas by adding sugar and cream. When well masticated the flavor is excellent and can not be improved by using dressings.

Be sure that the children have learned to masticate well before giving bananas, and then give only ripe ones. The flesh of the banana is so smooth and slippery that children often swallow it in big lumps, and then they frequently suffer.

Lemonade may be taken with fruit or flesh meals. As usually made it is quite nourishing, for it contains considerable sugar. Those who are troubled with sluggish liver may take it with benefit, but the less sugar used the better. Other fruit juices may be used likewise, but they should be fresh. If they are bottled, be sure that no fermentation is taking place in them. These juices may be served with the same kind of meals as lemonade. Most of them require dilution. Grape juice is very rich and a large glassful of the pure juice makes a good summer lunch. It should be sipped slowly. Those who like the combination may make a meal of fruit juice mixed with milk, half and half.

Grapes and strawberries, which are relished by most, disagree with some people. The skin of the Concord grape should be rejected, for it irritates many. If they are relished, the skins of most fruits may be eaten. When peeled apples lose a part of their flavor.

Olives are generally eaten pickled. The fruit in its natural state tastes very disagreeable to most people. The ripe olive is superior in flavor to the green, which is not usually relished at first.

The sweet fruits, by which we mean dried currants, raisins, figs and dates, and bananas should be classed with them, serve the body in the same way as do the breadstuffs, and may be substituted for starches at any time. They may be eaten at all seasons of the year, but are used most during cold weather. A moderate amount of them may be eaten with breadstuffs, or they may be taken alone, or with milk, or with nuts, or with acid fruit. They are very nourishing so it does not take much of them to make a meal. To get the full benefit, masticate thoroughly. They contain sugar in its best form, sugar that not impoverished by being deprived of its salts. Grape sugar needs very little preparation before it enters the blood. Starch and sugar are of equal value as nourishment. It seems that the sugar is available for energy sooner than the starch. Americans generally weary quickly of sweet foods, though they consume enormous quantities of refined sugar, but in tropical countries figs and dates are staple in many places and the inhabitants relish them day in and day out as we relish some of out staples. It is a matter of habit. Those who do not surfeit themselves do not weary quickly of any particular article of diet.

PREPARATION

Most fruits are best raw. Then their acids and salts are in their most available form. Those who become uncomfortable after eating acid fruit may know that they have abused their digestive organs and they should take it as an indication to reduce their food intake, simplify their diet, masticate better and eat more raw food. Those who overeat of starch or partake of much alcohol cultivate irritable stomachs, which object to the bracing fruit juices.

For the sake of a change fruits may be cooked. The more plainly they are cooked the better. Always use sugar in moderation, no matter whether the fruit is to be stewed or baked.

To stew fruit, clean and if necessary peel. Stew in sufficient water until tender. When almost done add what sugar is needed. When stewed thus less sugar is required than if the sweetening is done at the start.

Stewed fruit can be sweetened by adding raisins, figs or dates. This is relished by many. Figs and dates stewed by themselves are too sweet for many tastes. This can be remedied by making a sauce of figs or dates with tart apples or any other acid fruit that appeals in such combinations.

Baked apple: Place whole apples in large, deep pan; add about one-third cup of water and one and one-half teaspoonfuls sugar to each apple. Put into oven and bake until skins burst and the apples are well done. Serve with all the juice.

Boiled apple: Place whole apples in a stewing pan; add two teaspoonfuls sugar and one cup or more of water to each apple; use less sugar if desired. Cover the vessel tightly and boil moderately until the skins burst and the apples are well done.

All stewed fruits should be well done. Avoid making the fruit sauces too sweet.

Stewed prunes: A good prune needs no sweetening. Stew until tender. It is a good plan to let the prunes soak a few hours before stewing them. Raisins may be treated in the same way.

Prunes may be washed and put into a dish; then add hot water enough to about half cover them; cover the dish very tightly and put aside over night. The prunes need no further preparation before being eaten. If the covering is not tight it will be necessary to use more water. Raisins and sundried figs may be treated in the same way.

Unfortunately, most of our dried fruit is sulphured. Sulphurous acid fumes are employed, and you may be sure that this does the fruit no good. If you can get unsulphured fruit, do so. The sulphuring process is popular because it acts as a preservative and it is profitable because it allows the fruit to retain more water without spoiling than would be possible otherwise.

Canning fruit: It is very easy to can fruit, but it requires care. Select fruit that is not overripe. The work room should be clean and so should the cans and covers. It is not sufficient to rinse the cans in clean water. Both the jars and the covers should be taken from boiling water immediately before being used.

Use only sound fruit, cook it sufficiently, adding the sugar when the fruit is almost done. If you cook the fruit in syrup, do not have a heavy syrup. Put into jar while piping hot, filling the jar as full as possible, put on the cover immediately, turning until it fits snugly; turn jar upside down for a few hours to see if it leaks; tighten again and put in cool place.

An even better way, especially for berries, is to fill the jar with fruit, pour syrup over them, put the jars into a receptacle containing water and let this water boil until the berries are done; then fill the jars properly and seal. Some berries that lose their color when cooked in syrup retain it when treated this way.

Canned fruits are not as good as the fresh ones, but better than none. Be sure that they are not fermenting when opened. When proper care is exercised a spoiled jar is a rarity. If there is any doubt about the fruit, scald and cool before using. This destroys the ferments.

Fresh fruit is the best. Next comes fruit recently stewed or baked. If other fruit can not be obtained, get good dried fruit and stew it.

COMBINATIONS.

Fruits may be combined with almost any food, except that which is rich in starch, and even that combination may be used occasionally, although it is not the best. I have seen people who were supposed to be incurable get well when their breakfasts were mostly apple sauce and toast. However, sick people should avoid such combining entirely and healthy ones most of the time. Breakfasting on cereals and fruit is a mistake. Those who eat thus may say that they feel no bad results, but time will tell. Nowhere in our manner of feeding does nature demand of a healthy human being that he walk the chalk line. All she asks is that he be reasonable. So if you feel fine and want a shortcake for dinner take it. But the shortcake should be the meal, not the end of one that has already furnished too much food.

Fruit combines well with both milk and cheese. The impression to the contrary that has been gained from both medical and lay writers is due to false deductions based on premises not founded on facts. Milk and fruit, and nothing else, make very good meals in summer.

Fruit salads: A great variety of these salads can be made. Take two or three of the juicy fruits, slice and mix. Dress with a little sugar, or salt and olive oil, or simply olive oil, or no dressing. Some like a dressing of sour cream or of cottage cheese rather well thinned out. Raisins and other sweet fruits may also be used. Ripe banana may be one of the ingredients.

Such a salad may be eaten with a flesh or nut meal, or it may be used as a meal by itself. Fruit and cottage cheese make a meal that is both delicious and nourishing. A fruit salad strewed with nuts does the same.

Strawberries and sliced tomatoes dressed with cottage cheese make a good meal.

Lettuce, celery and tomatoes may be used in fruit salads.

A few fruit salads to serve as examples are: Apples, grapes and lettuce; peaches, strawberries and celery; bananas, pineapples and nuts; strawberries, tomatoes and lettuce. Combine to suit taste and dress likewise, but avoid large quantities of cream and sugar, not only on your salads, but on all fruits. No acid should be necessary, but if it is desired, use lemon juice or incorporate oranges as a part of the salad.

CHAPTER XVII.

OILS AND FATS.

Oils and fats are the most concentrated foods we have. Weight for weight, they contain more than twice as much fuel or energy value as any other food. Taken in moderation they are easily digested, but if taken in excess they become a burden to the system. About 7 or 8 per cent of the weight of a normal body is fat, and this fat is formed chiefly from the fatty foods taken into the system, supplemented by the sugar and starch.

When the body becomes very fat, it is a disease, called obesity. Fat people are never healthy. The fat usurps the place that should be occupied by normal tissues and organs. It crowds the heart and the lungs, and even replaces the muscle cells in the heart. The result is that the heart and lungs are overcrowded and overworked and the blood gets insufficient oxygen. Not only the lungs pant for breath after a little exercise, but the entire body. Much fat is as destructive of health as it is of beauty. Those who find themselves growing corpulent should decrease their intake of concentrated foods and increase their physical activity.

Our chief sources of fat supply are cream and butter, vegetable oils, nuts and the flesh of animals. Most meats, especially when mature, contain considerable fat. When the fat is mixed in with the meat, it is more difficult to digest than the lean flesh. Fresh fish, most of which contains very little fat, is digested very easily, while the fattest of all flesh, pork, is tedious of digestion.

There is an instinctive craving for fat with foods that contain little or none of it. That is why we use butter with cereals and lean fish, and oil dressings on vegetables. In moderation this is all right. Fats are not very rich in salts, which must be supplied by other foods.

Because of their great fuel value, more fats are naturally consumed in cold than in hot climates. The Esquimeaux thrive when a large part of their rations is fat. Such a diet would soon nauseate people in milder climes.

Fats and oils are used too much in cooking. Fried foods and those cooked in oil are made indigestible. Sometimes we read directions not to use animal fats, but to use olive oil or cotton seed oil for frying. It is poor cooking, no matter whether the grease is of animal or vegetable origin.

So far as food value and digestibility are concerned, there is no difference between animal and vegetable fats. Fresh butter is very good, and so is olive oil. Some vegetable oils contain indigestible substances. Cotton seed oil and peanut oil are much used. Sometimes they are sold in bottles under fancy lables as olive oil. The olive oils from California are fully as good as those imported from Spain, Italy and France and are more likely to be what is claimed for them than the foreign articles. In the past, much of our cotton seed oil has been bought by firms in southern Europe and sent back to us as fine olive oil! Such imposture is probably more difficult under our present laws than it was in the past.

Most oils become rancid easily and then are unfit for consumption. If taken in excess as food they have a splendid opportunity to spoil in the digestive tract, and then they help to poison the system. Taken in moderate quantities they are digested in the intestines and taken into the blood by way of the lymphatics. They may be stored in the body for a while, but finally they are burned, giving up much heat and energy.

Taking oils between meals as medicine or for fattening purposes is folly. People get all they need to eat in their three daily meals. Lunching is to be condemned.

CHAPTER XVIII.

MILK AND OTHER DAIRY PRODUCTS.

	Water	Protein	Fat	Carbohydrates	Ash	Calories per lb.
Whole milk	87.00	3.3	4.0	5.0	0.7	325
Cream	74.00	2.5	18.5	4.5	0.5	910
Buttermilk	91.00	3.0	0.5	4.8	0.7	165
Butter						

.... 82.4 ... ... 3475 Cheese, whole milk 33.70 26.0 34.2 2.3 3.8 1965 " skimmed milk 45.70 31.5 16.4 2.2 4.2 1320 --- -----------------------

The dairy products vary greatly. Some cows give richer milk than others. Butter may be almost pure fat, or it may contain much water and salt. The cheeses are rich or poor in protein and fats according to method of making. Cottage cheese may be well drained or quite watery. Therefore, this table gives only approximate contents.

Milk is not a beverage. It is a food. A quart of milk contains as much food and fuel value as eight eggs or twelve ounces of lean beef. That is, a cupful (one-half of a pint) is equal to two eggs or three ounces of lean beef. This shows that milk should not be taken to quench thirst, but to supply nourishment. Milk is one of our most satisfactory and economical albuminous foods, even at the present high prices. In many foods from 5 to 10 per cent of the protein goes to waste. In milk the waste does not ordinarily amount to more than about 1 per cent. This fluid generally leaves the stomach within one or one and one-half hours after being ingested.

In spite of its merits as a food some writers on dietetics advocate that adults stop using it, giving it only to the young.

Milk is an excellent food when properly used. When abused it tends to cause discomfort, disease and death, and so does every other food known to man. Milk is given in fevers and in other diseases, when the digestive and assimilative processes are suspended. This is a serious mistake and has caused untold numbers of deaths. When the digestion has gone on a strike all feeding is destructive. Milk and meat broths, which are generally given, are about the worst foods that could be selected under the circumstances, for they decay very easily, and are excellent food for the numerous bacteria that thrive in the digestive tract during disease. These foods must decay when they are not digested, for the internal temperature of the body during fevers is over one hundred degrees Fahrenheit.

When bacteria are present in excess they give off considerable poison, which makes the patient worse. If circumstances are such that it is necessary to feed during acute disease, which is always injurious to the patient, let the food be the least harmful obtainable, such as fruit juices. Even they do harm.

In our country cow's milk is used almost exclusively, and that is the variety that will be discussed in this chapter. In other lands the milk of the mare, the ass, the sheep, the goat and of other animals is used. Human milk is discussed in detail in the chapter on Infancy.

The objection voiced against cow's milk is that it is an unnatural food for man, only fit for the calf, which is equipped with several stomachs and is therefore able to digest the curds which are larger and tougher than the curds formed from human milk. It is said that the curds of cow's milk are so indigestible that the human stomach can not prepare them for entry into the blood. This is probably true, but it is also true of other protein-bearing foods. The digestion and assimilation of proteins are begun in the stomach and completed in the intestines, and the protein in milk is one of the most completely utilized of all proteins.

To call a food unnatural means nothing, for we can call nearly all foods unnatural and defend our position. A natural food is presumably a nutritious and digestible aliment that is produced in the locality where it is consumed, one that can be utilized without preparation or preservation. So we may say that a resident of New York should not use figs, dates, bananas and other products of tropical and semi-tropical climates, for they are not natural in the latitude of New York. We can take the position that it is unnatural for people to eat grains, which need much grinding, for the birds are the only living beings supplied with mills (gizzards). We can further say that it is unnatural to eat all cooked and baked foods. But such talk is not helpful. The more a person uses his brain the less power he has left for digestion and therefore it is necessary to prepare some of the foods so that they will be easy to digest. Man is such an adaptable creature that we are not sure what he subsisted on before he became civilized and are therefore unable to say what his natural food is. We know that in the tropics fruits play an important part in nourishing savages, while in the frozen north fat flesh is the chief food. Perhaps there is no natural food for man.

Some of those who advocate the disuse of milk have a substitute or imitation to take its place, nut milk made from finely ground nuts and water. Like all other imitations, it is inferior to the original. It is more difficult to digest than real milk and the flavor is quite different.

The objection that milk is indigestible is not borne out by the experience of those who give it under proper conditions. It is true that milk disagrees with a few, but so do such excellent foods as eggs, strawberries and Concord grapes, and many other aliments which are not difficult to digest. This is a matter of individual peculiarity. Some can take boiled milk, but are unable to take it fresh, and vice versa. Outside of the few exceptions, milk digests in a reasonable time and quite completely. It is easier to digest than the legumes (peas, beans, lentils) which are rich in protein. It is also easier to digest than nuts, which contain much protein. The milk sugar causes no trouble and cream is one of the easiest forms of fat to digest, if taken in moderation. The protein in milk will cause no inconvenience if the milk is eaten slowly, in proper combinations and not to excess. The rennet in the stomach curdles the casein. The hydrochloric acid and the pepsin in the gastric juice then begin to break down and dissolve the clots, and the process of digestion is completed in the small intestines.

Those who overeat of milk in combination with other foods will derive benefit from omitting the milk. They will also be benefitted if they continue using milk and omit either the starch or the meat. When foods disagree, in nearly every instance it is due to the fact that too much has been eaten and too many varieties partaken of at a meal. Some may single out the milk or the meat as the offenders. Others may point to the starches, and still others to the vegetables with their large amount of indigestible residue. They are all right and all wrong, for all the foods help to cause the trouble. However, such reasoning does not solve the problem. If the meals cause discomfort and disease, reduce the amount eaten, take fewer varieties at a meal and simplify the cooking. Those who eat simple meals and are moderate are not troubled with indigestion.

Those who eat such mushy foods as oatmeal and cream of wheat usually take milk or cream and sugar with them. This should not be done, for such dressing stimulates the appetite and leads to undermastication. Neither children nor adults chew these soft starchy foods enough. The result is that the breakfast ferments in the alimentary tract. After a few months or years of such breakfasts, some kind of disease is sure to develop. Mushy starches dressed with rich milk and sugar are responsible for a large per cent. of the so-called diseases of children, which are primarily digestive disturbances. Colds, catarrhs and adenoids are, of course, due to improper eating extending over a long period of time. Nothing should be eaten with mushy starches except a little butter and salt. After enough starch has been taken, a glass of milk may be eaten. If parents would only realize that they are jeopardizing the health and lives of their dear ones when they feed them habitually on these soft messes, which ferment easily, there would be a remarkable decrease in the diseases of childhood and in the disgraceful infant and childhood mortality, for several hundred thousand children perish annually in this country.

Milk is often referred to as a perfect food, and it is the perfect food for infants. The young thrive best on the healthy milk given by a female of their own species. Every baby should be fed at the breast. The milk contains the elements needed by the body.

The table at the head of this chapter shows that milk contains all essential aliments. The ash is composed of the various salts necessary for health, containing potassium, chlorine, calcium, magnesium, iron, silicon and other elements. For the nourishment of the body we need water, protein, fat, carbohydrates and salts, so it will be seen that milk is really a complete food. However, as the body grows the nutritive requirements change and milk is therefore not a balanced food for adults.

It may be interesting to note that there is no starch in milk and that infants fed at the breast exclusively obtain no starchy food. Many babies get no starch for nine, ten or even twelve months, and this is well, for they do not need it. They grow and flourish best without it.

Milk is an emulsion. It is made up of numerous tiny globules floating in serum. The size of the globules varies, but the average is said to be about 1/10,000 of an inch in diameter. These globules are fatty bodies. There are other small bodies, containing protein and fat, which have independent molecular movement. The milk is a living fluid. When it is tampered with it immediately deteriorates. Without doubt, nature intended that the milk should go directly from the mammary gland into the mouth of the consumer, but this is not practicable when we take it away from the calf. However, if we are to use sweet milk it is best to consume it as nearly like it is in its natural state as possible.

It is quite common to drink milk rapidly. This should not be done. Take a sip or a spoonful at a time and move it about in the mouth until it is mixed with saliva. It is not necessary to give it as much mouth preparation as is given to starchy food. If it is drunk rapidly like water large curds from in the stomach. If it is insalivated it coagulates in smaller curds and is more easily digested, for the digestive juices can tear down small soft curds more easily than the large tough ones.

Milk should not form a part of any meal when other food rich in protein is eaten. Our protein needs are small, and it is easy to get too much. Whole wheat bread and milk contain all the nourishment needed. On such a diet we can thrive indefinitely. This is information, not a recommendation. The bread should be eaten either before or after partaking of the milk. Do not break the bread into the milk. If this is done, mastication will be slighted. Bread needs much mastication and insalivation. When liquid is taken with the bread, the saliva does not flow so freely as when it is eaten dry.

Fruit and milk make a good combination, but no starchy foods are to be taken in this meal. Take a glass of milk, either sweet or sour, and what fruit is desired, insalivating both the fruit and the milk thoroughly. If you have read that the combination of fruit and milk has proved fatal, rest assured that those who made such reports only looked at the surface, for other foods and other influences were having their effects on the system. Many people die of food-poisoning and apoplexy. These bad results are due to wrong eating covering a long period and it is folly to blame the last meal. It would be queer if fruit and milk were not occasionally a part of the last meal.

In winter, figs, dates or raisins with milk make an excellent lunch or breakfast. These fruits take the place of bread, for though they are not starchy, they contain an abundance of fruit sugar, which is more easily digested than the starch. Starch must be converted into sugar before the system can use it.

On hot days milk and acid fruit make a satisfying meal. Many believe that milk and acid fruit should not be taken in the same meal, because the acid curdles the milk. As we have already seen, the milk must be curdled before it can be digested. If this step in digestion is performed by the acid in the fruit no more harm is done than when it is performed by the lactic acid bacteria. Fruit juices and milk do not combine to form deadly poisons. If fruit and milk are eaten in moderation and no other food is taken at that meal the results are good. However, if fruit, milk, bread, meat, cake and pickles make up the meal, the results may be bad. Such eating is very common. But do not blame the fruit and the milk when the whole meal is wrong.

Likewise, if a hearty meal has been eaten and before this has had time to digest a lunch is made of fruit and milk, trouble may ensue. All the foods may be good, but a time must come when the body will object to being overfed. In summertime much less food is needed than during the cold months. Nevertheless, barring the Christmas holidays and Thanksgiving, people overeat more in summer than at any other time of the year. Picnics often degenerate into stuffing matches. We should expect many cases of serious illness to follow them, and such is the case.

Sometimes the milk is so carelessly handled that it becomes poisonous and at other times the fruit is tainted, but generally bad combinations and overeating are the factors that cause trouble when the fruit and milk combination is blamed.

Buttermilk and clabbered milk are more easily digested by many than is the fresh milk. In Europe sour milk is a more common food than in this country. Here many do not know how excellent it is. Two glasses of milk, or less, make a good warm-weather lunch.

Those who have a tendency to be bilious should use cream very sparingly. Bilious people always overeat, otherwise their livers would not be in rebellion. The fat, in the form of cream, arouses decided protest on the part of overburdened livers.

A theory has found its way into dietetic literature, sometimes disguised as a truth, to the effect that boiled or hot milk is absorbed directly into the blood stream without being digested. This is contrary to everything we know about digestion and assimilation, and although it is a fine enough theory it does not work out in practice. I have seen bad results when nothing but a small amount of the hot milk was fed to patients with weak digestive power.

Perhaps others have had better results. When the system demands a rest from food, nothing but water should be given. Boiled or natural milk is then as bad as any other food, and worse than most, for in the absence of digestive power it soon becomes a foul mass, swarming with billions of bacteria. The system is compelled to absorb some of the poisons given off by the micro-organisms and the results are disastrous.

Every food we take must be modified by our bodies before entering the circulation, and milk is no exception.

When milk is allowed to stand for a while the sugar ferments, through the action of the lactic acid bacteria. The sugar is turned into lactic acid, which combines with the casein and when this process has continued for a certain length of time the result is clabbered milk or sour milk. The length of time varies with the temperature and the care given the milk. If milk remains sweet for a long time during warm weather, discharge the milkman and patronize one whose product sours more quickly, for milk that remains sweet has been subjected to treatment. All kinds of preservative treatment cause deterioration. If extraordinary care is taken with the milk and it is kept at a temperature of about forty-two degrees Fahrenheit, it may remain sweet five or six weeks, provided it is not exposed to the air, but such care is at present not practicable in commercial dairies. The milk contains unorganized ferments which spoil it in time without exposure to bacterial influences. These ferments cause digestion or decay of the milk.

Fresh butter is a palatable form of fat, which digests easily. Like all other milk products, it must be kept clean and cold, or it will soon spoil. Butter absorbs other flavors quickly and should therefore not be placed near odorous substances. It is best unsalted and in Europe it is very commonly served thus. When people learn to demand unsalted butter they will get good butter, for no one can palm off oleomargarine or other imitations under the guise of fresh unsalted butter. Unsalted butter must be fresh or it will be refused by the nose and the palate. Salt and other preservatives often conceal age and corruption of foods.

Butter combines well with starches and vegetables, in fact, it can be used in moderation with any other food, when the body needs fat. Butter should not be used to cook starches or proteins in. Greasy cooking should be banished from our kitchens.

Milk is a complex food, highly organized, and therefore is easily injured or spoiled. The general rule is that the more complex a food is, the more easily it spoils. It is rather difficult at present to get wholesome milk enough to supply the people of our large cities. When it is boiled, the milk keeps longer, but boiled milk is spoiled milk. The fine flavor is lost, the casein, which is the principal protein of milk, is toughened, the milk, which is normally a living liquid, is killed, the chemical balance is lost, the organic salts being rendered partly inorganic. Milk that is unfit to eat without being boiled is not fit to eat afterwards, for the poisonous end products of bacterial life remain.

The milk is soured by the bacteria it contains. The lactic acid bacteria are harmless. When there is a lack of care and cleanliness, other bacteria get into the milk, and these are also harmless to people in good health, and most of them are not injurious to sick people. The bacteria (germs) do not cause disease, but when disease has been established, they offer their kindly offices as scavengers. Bacteria thrive in sick people, especially when they are fed when digestive power is lacking. Boiling retards the souring of milk, but when fat and protein are boiled together the protein becomes hard to digest. Milk is rich in both fat and protein. Excessive heat turns the milk brown, the milk sugar being carameled.

Babies do not thrive on boiled milk. They may look fat, but instead of having the desirable firmness of normal children, they are puffy. Children fed on denatured milk fall victims to diseases very easily, especially to diseases which are due to lack of organic salts, such as rickets and malnutrition.

Pasteurization of milk is very popular. This is objectionable for the same reasons that boiling is condemned, though not to the same extent. Pasteurization is heating the milk to about 140 to 150 degrees Fahrenheit. This kills many of the bacteria, but many escape and when the milk is cooled off they begin to multiply and flourish again. It is estimated that pasteurized milk contains one-fourth as many bacteria as natural milk. So nothing is gained, and the milk is partly devitalized. The advocates of pasteurization give statistics showing that milk so treated has been instrumental in decreasing infant mortality. But please bear in mind that previously a great deal of milk unfit for consumption was fed to the babies. Those who pasteurize milk generally are careful enough to see that they get a good product in the first place.

If we can't get good milk we can do without it, for it is not a necessary food, but we can get good milk if we make the effort. If the milk is filthy, boiling or pasteurizing does not remove the dirt. Gauthier says of pasteurization: "Sometimes it is heated up to 70 degrees (Centigrade) with pressure of carbonic acid. But even in this case pasteurization does not destroy all germs, particularly those of tuberculosis, peptonizing bacteria of cowdung, and the dust of houses and streets, etc."

Even boiling does not kill the spores of bacteria unless it is continued until the milk is rendered entirely unfit for food. To kill these spores it is necessary to boil the milk several times. The spores are small round or oval bodies which form within the bacterial envelope when these micro-organisms are subjected to unfavorable conditions. The spores resist heat and cold that would kill almost any other form of life. When conditions are favorable they develop into bacteria again.

After heating, the cream does not rise so quickly nor does it separate so completely as it does in natural milk. This is due to the toughening of the casein in the milk.

Heating partly disorganizes the delicately balanced salts contained in the milk. The result is that they can not be utilized so easily and completely by the body, for the human organism demands its food in an organic state, that is, in the condition built up by vegetation or by animals. We may consume iron filings and remain anemic, in fact, the effect the iron medication has is to ruin the teeth, digestive organs and other parts of the body as a consequence. But if we partake of such foods as apples, cabbage, lettuce and spinach, the necessary salt is taken into the blood.

Heating milk also makes it constipating. True, normal people can take boiled milk without becoming constipated, but how many normal people are there? We are sorely enough afflicted in this way now. Let us have a supply of natural milk or go without it. It is not my desire to convey the impression that it does any harm to scald or boil milk occasionally, but if done daily it does harm, especially to the young. Scalded milk has its proper place in dietetics.

Occasionally we find a person who has persistent chronic diarrhea. If he is in condition to eat anything, this annoying affliction is usually overcome in a reasonable time if the patient will take boiled or scalded milk in moderation three times a day, and nothing else except water.

How are we to obtain good milk? We can do it by using common sense, care and cleanliness.

It is well to remember that there are bacteria in all ordinary milk, and that if the milk is from healthy cows and is kept clean and cold these bacteria are harmless. Most of them are the lactic acid bacteria, which change the milk sugar into acid. When the milk has attained a certain degree of acidity, the lactic acid bacteria are unable to thrive and the souring process is slowed up and finally stopped. Most of the other bacteria in milk perish when lactic acid is formed. This is why stale sweet milk is often harmful, when the same kind of milk allowed to sour can be taken with impunity.

If the milk is kept in a cold place the bacteria multiply slowly. If it is kept in a warm place they increase in numbers at a rate that is marvelous, and consequently the milk sours much sooner. Even if the milk is kept cold, bacterial growth will soon take place, but it will perhaps not be lactic acid bacteria. It may be a form that causes the milk to become ropy and slimy or one that gives it a bad odor.

Bacteria are like other forms of vegetation, such as grass, weeds, flowers and trees, in that some flourish best under one condition and others under dissimilar conditions, and they struggle one against the other for subsistence and existence. Like flowers there are thousands of different forms of bacteria and they vary according to their food and environment.

Peculiar odors in milk generally come from certain kinds of food given to the cows, such as turnips; from bacterial action; or from flavors absorbed from other foods or from odors in the air. Milk should not be exposed to odorous substances, for it becomes tainted very quickly. Sometimes yeast finds its way into milk and causes decomposition of the sugar with the formation of carbon dioxide and alcohol.

A count of the bacteria in milk often serves a good purpose, for it shows whether it is good and has had proper care. The consumers have a right to demand milk low in bacteria, for if no preservatives have been used, that means clean milk. If we could live in our pristine state of beatific bliss, if such it was, we would not have to use milk after childhood is past, but our present condition demands the use of easily digested foods and to many milk is almost a necessity.

The milk in the udder of a healthy cow is almost surely free from bacteria, but the moment it is exposed to the air these little beings start to drop into the fluid.

The bacterial standards given by various city health departments vary. Those who are mathematically inclined may find the following figures interesting: In some great cities they allow 500,000 bacteria to the cubic centimeter of milk. A cubic centimeter contains about twenty-five drops. In other words, they allow 20,000 bacteria per drop. This may seem very lively milk, but these bacteria are so small that about 25,000 of them laid end to end measure only about an inch, and it would take 17,000,000,000,000 of them to weigh an ounce, according to estimates. These are the tiny vegetables we hear and read so much about, that we are warned against and fear so much. Truly the pygmies are having their innings and making cowards of men. The bacteria multiply by the simple process of growing longer and splitting into two, fission, as it is called, and the process is so rapid that within an hour or two after being formed a bacterium may be raising a family of its own.

Some of the milk brought to the cities contains as many as 15,000,000 bacteria per cubic centimeter, that is, about 600,000 per drop. This milk is either very filthy or it has been poorly cared for and should not be given to babies and young children. The filthiest milk may contain several billion bacteria to the cubic centimeter.

By using care milk containing but 100, or even fewer, bacteria per drop can be produced. From the standpoint of cleanliness this is excellent milk. Of course, the dairyman who takes pride enough in his work to produce such milk will sell nothing but what is first-class, and if he has business acumen he can always get more than the market price for his product.

The talk about germs has been overdone, but no one can deny that the study of bacteriology has made people more careful about foods. The filthy dairies that were the rule a few years ago are slowly being replaced by dairies that are comfortable, well lighted and clean. Do not allow the germs to scare you, for if ordinary precautions are taken no more of them will be present than are necessary, and they are necessary. They thrive best in filth, and they are dangerous only to those who live so that they have no resistance.

Wholesome milk can be produced only by healthy animals. Bovine health can be secured by the same means as human health. The cows must be properly fed and housed. They must have both ventilation and light. They must not be unduly worried. If a nursing of an angry mother's milk is at times poisonous enough to kill a baby, you may be sure that the milk from an abused, irritated and angry cow is also injurious. If the animals are kept comfortable and happy they will do the best producing, both in quality and quantity. It may sound far-fetched to some to advocate keeping animals happy in order to get them to produce much and give quality products, but it is good science and good sense. Happy cows give more and better milk than the mistreated ones. The singing hens are the best layers.

Cows should have fresh green food all the year, and this can be obtained in winter time by using silage. It is a mistake to give cows too much of concentrated foods, such as oil meals and grains. Cattle can not long remain well on exclusive rations of too heating and stimulating foods. When fed improperly they soon fall prey to various diseases, such as rheumatism and tuberculosis. It is the same with other domestic animals. The horse when overfed on grain develops stiff joints. The hogs that are compelled to live exclusively on concentrated, heating rations are liable to die of cholera. Young turkeys that have nothing but corn and wheat to eat die in great numbers from the disease known as blackhead. It is the same law running all through nature, applying to the high and to the low, that improper nourishment brings disease and death.

When cattle roam wild, the green grasses (sundried in winter) are their principal source of food. Man should be careful not to deviate too much, for forced feeding is as harmful to animals as it is to man.

The following excellent recommendations for the care of milk are given by Dr. Charles E. North of the New York City Milk Commission:

"No coolers, aerators, straining cloths or strainers should be used.

"The hot milk should be taken to the creamery as soon as possible.

"The night's milk should be placed in spring or iced water higher than the milk on the inside of the can. It should not be stirred, and the top of the can should be open a little way to permit ventilation.

"The milking pails and cans will be sterilized and dried at the creamery, and should be carefully protected until they are used.

"Brush the udder and wipe with a clean cloth; wash with clean water and dry with a clean towel.

"Whitewash the cow stable at least twice yearly.

"Feed no dusty feed until after milking.

"Remove all manure from cow stable twice daily.

"Keep barnyard clean and have manure pile at least 100 feet from the stable.

"Have all stable floors of cement, properly drained.

"Have abundant windows in cowstables to permit sunlight to reach the floor.

"Arrange a proper system of ventilation.

"Do not use milk from any cows suspected of gargot or of any udder inflammation. Such milk contains enormous numbers of bacteria.

"Brush and groom cows from head to foot as horses are groomed.

"Use no dusty bedding; wood shavings or sawdust give least dust.

"Use an abundance of ice in water tank for cooling milk."

Perhaps some will take issue with the doctor on the first paragraph of his recommendation. If straining cloths are used they should be well rinsed in tepid water, washed and then boiled. However, if his recommendations are carried out in letter and spirit no straining is necessary.

Herr Klingelhofer near Dusseldorf, Germany., runs a model dairy. The cows, stables, milkers, containers, in fact, all things connected with the dairy are scrupulously clean. The milkers do not even touch the milk stools, carrying them strapped to their backs. The milk is strained through sterilized cotton and cooled.

The cows are six and seven years old and are milked for ten or twelve months and they are not bred during this time. The first part of the milk drawn from each teat is not used, for that part is not clean, containing dirt and bacteria.

This milk is practically free from bacteria, for without adding preservatives it will remain sweet, for as long as thirteen days. If ordinary milk fails to sour in two or three days it shows that it has been treated.

According to the Country Gentleman, it will cost from one cent and a quarter to one cent and three-quarters extra per quart to produce clean milk. Healthy adults can take milk teeming with bacteria without harm, but for babies it is best to have very few or none in the milk. At Dusseldorf the babies used to die as they do here when fed unclean milk. Herr Klingelhofer says that when fed on his product "sterben keine." (None die.)

This is submitted to those who advocate pasteurizing the milk. Denatured milk makes sickly babies. Clean natural milk makes healthy babies. The extra cost of less than two cents a quart is not prohibitive. Most fathers, no matter how poor, waste more than that daily on tobacco and alcoholics. The extra cost would be more than saved in lessened doctor bills, to say nothing of funeral expenses. The recompense that comes from the satisfaction of having thriving, sturdy, healthy children can not be figured in dollars and cents.

Dr. Robert Mond, of London, after investigating for years, has come to the conclusion that sterilized milk predisposes to tuberculosis, instead of preventing it. He believes that milk so treated is so inferior that he would not personally use it. That sterilized milk predisposes to tuberculosis, as well as to other diseases which can attack the body only when it is run down, is natural. Any food that has been rendered inferior can not build the robust health that comes to those who live on natural food. Adults who use sterilized milk should counteract its bad effects by partaking liberally of fresh fruits and vegetables.

If the milk is clean, put into clean containers by careful milkers and is then kept cold until delivered, it will reach the consumers in good condition. Do not let the fact that when you consume a glass of milk you are also engulfing some millions of bacteria bother you, for bacteria are necessary to our existence. If all the bacteria on earth should perish, it would also mean the end of the human race.

Today the progressive farmer is coming to the fore. He is a man who is justly proud of his work, so it will probably not be long before all city people who desire clean milk can get it.

The milk cure consists in feeding sick people on nothing but milk for varying periods. Generally the patient is told to either take great quantities three or four times a day, or to take smaller quantities perhaps every half hour. The milk cure has no special virtue, except that it is a monotonous diet. The body soon rebels if forced to subsist on an excessive amount of but one kind of food. The individual loses his desire for food and even becomes nauseated. If the advocates of the milk cure would prescribe milk in moderation, instead of in excess, they would have better success. (It is fully as harmful to partake of too much milk as it is to eat excessively of other foods.)

The benefit derived from the milk cure comes from the simplicity, not from the milk. A grape cure, an orange cure or a bread and milk cure would be as beneficial. The milk cure is ancient. It was employed twenty-five centuries ago.

Clabbered milk: Clabbered milk or sour milk needs no special preparation. Put the milk into an earthen or china dish. Do not use metal dishes, for the lactic acid acts upon various metals. Cover the dish so as to keep particles of matter in the air away, but the covering is not to be airtight. Put the dish in a warm place, but not in the sun. Milk that sours in the sun or in an air-tight bottle is generally of poor flavor. Clabbered milk is a good food. It does not form big, tough curds in the stomach, it is easy to digest, and the lactic acid helps to keep the alimentary tract sweet. The various forms of milk may be used in similar combinations.

Buttermilk: The real buttermilk is what remains of the cream after the fat has been removed by churning. It is slightly acid and has a characteristic taste, to most people very agreeable. The flavor is different from that of artificially made buttermilk. In composition it is almost like whole milk, except that it contains very little fat.

Many people make buttermilk by beating the clabbered milk thoroughly, until it becomes light. The buttermilk made from sweet milk and the various brands of bacterial ferments obtainable at the drug stores is all right. These ferments have as their basis the lactic acid bacteria, and if the manufacturers wish to call their germs by other names, such as Bacillus Bulgaricus, no harm is done. It is unnecessary to add any of these ferments, for the milk clabbers about as quickly without them.

Buttermilk is an excellent food. The casein can be seen in fine flakes in the real buttermilk. Adults usually digest buttermilk and clabbered milk more easily than the sweet milk. The lactic acid seems to be quite beneficial. Metchnikoff thought for a while that he had discovered how to ward off decay and old age by means of the lactic acid bacteria in milk.

Milk can be clabbered quickly by adding lemon juice to sweet milk.

Junket: Add rennet to milk and let it stand until it thickens. The milk is not to be disturbed while coagulation takes place, for agitation will cause a separation of the whey. The rennet can be bought at the drug stores.

Whey contains milk sugar, some salts, and a little albumin. It is easily digested, but not very nourishing. It is what is left of the milk after the fat and almost all of the protein are removed.

Cottage cheese: This is sometimes called Dutch cheese or white cheese. It is a delicious and nutritious dairy product that is easy to digest. Put the clabbered milk in a muslin bag, hang the bag up and allow the milk to lose its whey through drainage. In summer this bag must be kept in a cool place. After draining, beat the curds. Then add enough clabbered milk to make the curds soft when well beaten. A small amount of cream may also be added. Cottage cheese made in this way is superior in flavor and digestibility to that which has been scalded. No seasoning is needed. A little salt is allowable, but sugar and pepper should not be used. Fruit and cottage cheese make a satisfying as well as nutritious meal.

Delicious cottage cheese is also made by using the whole clabbered milk. Hang it up to drain in a bag until it has lost a part of its whey. Then beat it until the curds are rather small, but not fine. No milk or cream is to be added to this, for it contains all the fat that is in the whole milk. Do not drain this cheese so long that it becomes dry.

Other cheeses: The various cheeses on the market are made principally from ripened curds, with which more or less fat has been mixed. The ripening is a form of decay, and it is no exaggeration to say that some of the very ripe cheeses on the market are rotten. The flavors are due to ferments, molds and bacteria, which split up the proteins and the fats.

The mild cheeses are generally good and may be eaten with fruits or vegetables or with bread. Two or three ounces are sufficient for the protein part of the meal, taking the place of flesh. Use less if less is desired.

When cheese becomes very odorous and ripe, no one with normal nose and palate will eat it. People who partake of excessive amounts of meats or alcoholic beverages are often fond of these foul cheeses. One perversion leads to another.

Cheese of good quality, eaten in moderation, is a nutritious food, easily digested. Gauthier says of cheese: "Indeed, this casein, which has the composition of muscular tissue, scarcely produces during digestion either residue or toxins."

Because good cheese is concentrated and of agreeable flavor, it is necessary to guard against overeating. An excess of rich cheese soon causes trouble with the liver or constipation or both.

Cheese should not be eaten in the same meal with fish, meat, eggs, nuts or legumes, for such combining makes the protein intake too great. There is nothing incompatible about such combinations, but it is safest not to make them. The course dinners, ending up with a savory cheese, crackers and coffee, are abominations. They are health-destroyers. They lead to overeating. As nearly everybody overeats, and because overeating is the greatest single factor in producing disease and premature death, it is advisable not to eat cheese and other foods rich in protein in the same meal. The greater the variety of food, the more surely the diner will overeat.

The term, "full cream cheese" is misleading, for cheeses are not made of whole cream. The cream does not contain enough protein (casein) for the manufacture of cheese. Some cheeses are made of skimmed milk. Others are made of milk which contains part, or even all, of the cream. Some have cream added. The cheeses containing but a moderate amount of fat are the best.

The popular Roquefort cheese is made of a mixture of goat's milk and sheep's milk. The savor is due to bacterial action and fat saponification, which result in ammonia, glycerine, alcohol, fatty acids and other chemicals in very small quantities.

The peculiar colorings which run in streaks through some cheeses that are well ripened are due to molds, bacteria and yeasts. Gentlemen who would discharge the cook if a moldy piece of bread appeared on the table, eat decaying, moldy cheese with relish.

The best cheese of all is cottage cheese. People of normal taste will soon weary of the frequent consumption of strong cheese, but they can take cottage cheese every other day with relish. Occasionally put a few caraway seeds in it if this flavor is agreeable.

Cottage cheese may be eaten plain or with bread, or with fruit or vegetables. It may be used as dressing both on fruit and vegetable salads.

Cheese should play no part in the alimentation of the sick, with the exception of cottage cheese, which may be given to almost anyone who is in condition to eat anything. The other cheeses are too concentrated for sick people. In acute disease nothing is to be fed.

Skimmed milk is about the same in composition as buttermilk. It is inferior in flavor, but a good food. It is used a great deal in cooking. Milk should not be used very much in cooking. When cooked it does not digest very readily and it has a tendency to make other foods indigestible.

Sour cream or clabbered cream is best when it is taken from clabbered milk. It may be used as dressing on fruits and salads. Sweet cream will clabber, but it is not as delicious as when it clabbers on the milk.

Clotted cream is made by putting the milk aside in pans in a cool place until the cream rises. Then, without disturbing the cream, scald the milk. Put the pan aside until the contents are cold and remove the cream, which has a rich, agreeable flavor. This may be used as a dressing.

Whipped cream and ice cream are so familiar that they hardly need comment. Cream is such a rich food that it must be eaten in moderation. Otherwise it will cause discomfort and disease. Ice cream is made of milk and cream, in varying proportions, flavored to taste and frozen. It is not necessary to add eggs and cornstarch. If eaten slowly it is a good food, but taken in too large quantities and too rapidly it may cause digestive troubles. It is not best to chill the stomach. Those with weak digestion should be very careful not to do so.

Buttermilk is sometimes flavored and frozen. This ice is easy to digest. Some doctors recommend this dish to their convalescents. It is an agreeable change, and can be eaten by many who are unable to take care of the rich ice cream.

CHAPTER XIX.

MENUS.

For a balanced dietary we need some building food, protein; some force food, starch, sugar and fat; some of the mineral salts in organic form, best obtained from raw fruits and vegetables; and a medium in which the foods can be dissolved, water.

We need a replenishment of these food stuffs at intervals, but it is not necessary to take all of them at the same meal, or even during the same day. Those who believe that all alimentary principles must enter into every meal must necessarily injure themselves through too complex eating. In talking of these alimentary principles, reference is made to them only when they are present in appreciable quantities.

To have the subject better in hand, let us again classify the most important foods:

Flesh foods, which are rich in protein.

Nuts, which contain considerable protein and fat.

Milk and cheese, which contain much protein.

Eggs, taken principally for their protein.

Cereals, the most important contents being starches.

Tubers, containing much starch.

Legumes, rich in protein and starch.

Fresh fruits, well flavored and high in salt contents.

Sweet fruits, containing much fruit sugar.

Succulent vegetables, chiefly valuable because of salts and juices.

Fats and oils, no matter what their source, are concentrated foods which furnish heat and energy when burned in the body.

When people are free and active in the fresh air they can eat in a way that would soon ruin the digestive powers of those who lead more artificial lives. It is a well known fact that we can go hunting, fishing, tramping or picnicking and eat mixtures and quantities of foods that would ordinarily give us discomfort. The freedom and activity, the change and the better state of mind give greater digestive power.

Those who wish to live their best must pay some attention to the combination of food. It is true that very moderate people, those who take no more food than the body demands, can combine about as they please. These moderate people do not care to mix their foods much. They are satisfied with very plain fare. Much as we dislike to acknowledge the fact, nearly all of us take too much food, even those who most strongly preach moderation. By combining properly much of the harmful effect of overeating can be overcome.

FRUITARIANS.

I class as fruitarians those who eat only cereals, fruits and nuts. This may not be a correct definition, but after reading much literature on dietetics it is the best I can do. Their combinations should present no difficulties.

They should take cereals once or twice a day; nuts once or twice a day; fruit once a day in winter and once or twice a day in summer. The winter fruit should be sweet part of the time. In summer it can be the juicy fruit and berries at all times.

The fruitarians should be careful to avoid the habitual combination of acid fruits with their cereals.

One meal a day can be made of one or two varieties of fruit and nothing else. Nuts may be added to the fruit at times.

Another meal may be made of some cereal product with nut butter or some kind of vegetable oil.

A third meal may be some form of sweet fruit, with which may be eaten either bread or nuts, or better still, combine one sweet fruit with an acid one.

Most people would consider such a diet very limited, but it is easy to thrive on it, and it is not a tiresome one. There are so many varieties of fruits, nuts and cereals that it is easy to get variety. These foods do not become monotonous when taken in proper amounts. On such a diet it does not make much difference which meal is breakfast, lunch or dinner. The rule should be to take the heartiest meal after the heavy work is done, for hearty meals do not digest well if either mind or body is hard at work.

It is not difficult to get all the food necessary in two meals, but inasmuch as the three meal a day plan is prevalent the menus here given include that number of meals.

Breakfast: Apples, baked or raw.

Lunch: Brown rice and raisins.

Dinner: Whole wheat zwieback with nut butter.

Breakfast: Oranges or grapefruit.

Lunch: Pecans and figs.

Dinner: Bread made of rye or whole wheat flour, with nut butter or olive oil.

Breakfast: Any kind of berries.

Lunch: Dates.

Dinner: Whole wheat bread, with or without oil, Brazil nuts.

These combinations are indeed simple, but these foods are very nourishing and most of them concentrated, so it is best not to mix too much. They are natural foods, which digest easily when taken in moderation, but if eaten to excess they soon produce trouble.

It is no hardship to live on simple combinations. We have so much food that we have fallen into the bad habit of partaking of too great variety at a meal. The fact is that those who combine simply enjoy their foods more than those who coax their appetite with too great variety. There is no physical hardship connected with simple eating, and as soon as the mind is made up to it, neither is there any mental hardship.

VEGETARIANS.

It is difficult to give an acceptable definition for vegetarianism. For a working basis we shall take it for granted that those are vegetarians who reject flesh foods. Those who wish can also reject dairy products and eggs. It is largely a matter of satisfying the mind.

The chief trouble with the vegetarians is that they believe that the fact that they abstain from flesh will bring them health. So they combine all kinds of foods and take several kinds of starches and fruits at the same meal. The consequence is that they soon get an acid condition of the digestive organs and a great deal of fermentation. Among vegetarians, prolapsus of the stomach and bowels is quite common, and this is due to gas pressure displacing the organs.

Their foods are all right, but their combinations, as a rule, are bad. The various vegetarian roasts, composed of nuts, cereals, legumes and succulent vegetables are hard to digest. It would be much better for them not to make such dishes.

A few suggestions for vegetarian combining follow:

Breakfast: Berries and a glass of milk.

Lunch: Baked potatoes and lettuce with oil.

Dinner: Nuts, cooked succulent vegetables, one or two varieties, sliced tomatoes.

Breakfast: Cottage cheese and oranges.

Lunch: Nuts and raisins.

Dinner: Whole wheat bread, stewed onions, butter, salad of lettuce and celery.

Breakfast: Cantaloupe.

Lunch: Buttermilk, bread and butter.

Dinner: Nuts, stewed succulent vegetables, lettuce and sliced tomatoes, with or without oil.

Breakfast: Boiled brown rice with raisins and milk.

Lunch: Grapes.

Dinner: Cooked lentils or baked beans, lettuce and celery.

OMNIVOROUS PEOPLE.

In this country, most people are omnivorous. The food is plentiful and people believe in generous living. They put upon their tables at each meal enough variety for a whole day and the custom is to eat some of each. Some breakfasts are heavy enough for dinners. Three heavy meals a day are common. Some can eat this way for years and be in condition to work most of the time, but they are never 100 per cent. efficient. They are never as able as they could be. Besides, they have their times of illness and grow old while they should be young. They generally die while they should be in their prime, leaving their friends and families to mourn them when they ought to be at their best. They are worn out by their food supply, plus other conventional bad habits.

One of the best plans that has been proposed for omnivorous people is that which has been worked out by Dr. J. H. Tilden. Its skeleton is, fruit once a day, starchy food once a day, flesh or other protein with succulent vegetables once a day. I shall make up menus for a few days based on this plan:

Breakfast: Baked apples, a glass of milk.

Lunch: Boiled rice with butter.

Dinner: Roast mutton, spinach and carrots, salad of raw vegetables.

Breakfast: Cantaloupe.

Lunch: Biscuits or toast with butter, buttermilk.

Dinner: Pecans, two stewed succulent vegetables, salad of lettuce, tomatoes and cucumbers, dressing.

Breakfast: Peaches, cottage cheese.

Lunch: Baked potatoes, butter, lettuce.

Dinner: Fresh fish baked, liberal helping of one, two or three of the raw salad vegetables.

Breakfast: Shredded wheat or puffed wheat sprinkled with melted butter, glass of milk.

Lunch: Watermelon.

Dinner: Roast beef, boiled cabbage, stewed onions, butter dressing, sliced tomatoes with salt and oil.

The doctor allows considerable dessert. That generally goes with the dinner.

It is nonsense to write, "So and so shalt thou eat and not otherwise." The menus here given simply serve as suggestions. Where one succulent vegetable is mentioned another may be substituted. One cereal may be substituted for another. One juicy fruit for another. One sweet fruit for another. One legume for another. One food rich in protein for another.

In combining food the principal things to remember are:

Use only a few foods at a meal; use only one hearty, concentrated food in a meal, as a rule, with the exception that various fats and oils in moderation are allowable as dressings for fruits, vegetables and starches; that much fat or oil retards the digestion of the rest of the food; that the habitual combining of acid food with foods heavy in starch is a trouble-maker; that concentrated starchy foods should be taken not to exceed twice a day; that the heating, stimulating foods rich in protein, which include nearly all meats, should be taken only once a day in winter, and less in summer; that either raw fruit or raw vegetables should be a part of the daily food intake, because the salts they contain are essential to health; that fats should be used sparingly in summer, but more freely in winter; that juicy fruits are to be used liberally in summer and sparingly in winter, when the sweet fruits are to take their place a part of the time.

The dried sweet fruits are quite different from the fresh juicy ones. The former serve more the purpose of the starches than that of fruits. They are rich in sugar, which produces heat and energy. The same is true of the banana, which is about one-fifth sugar. It is not as sweet as would be expected from this fact. Some sugars are sweeter than others. This you can easily verify by tasting some milk sugar and then taking the same amount of commercial sugar made of cane or beets.

The food need in summer is surprisingly small, so small that the average person will scarcely believe it. Some writers on dietetics advise eating as much in summer as in winter. How they can do so it is difficult to understand, for reason tells us that in summertime practically no food is needed for heating purposes, and that is how most of the food is used. A little experience and experiment show that reason is right. Nature herself confirms this fact, for at the tropics she has made it easy for man to subsist on fruits, while in the polar regions she furnishes him the most heating of all foods, fats.

Because fats are so concentrated it is very easy to take too much of them. An ounce of butter contains as much nourishment as about twenty-five ounces of watermelon. Those who simplify their cooking and their combining and partake of food in moderation are repaid many times over in improved health. It is necessary to supply good building material in proper form if we would have health.

CHAPTER XX.

DRINK.

There is but one real beverage and that is water. The other so-called beverages are foods, stimulants or sedatives. Milk is a rich food, one glass having as much food value as two eggs. Coffee, tea, chocolate and cocoa are stimulants, with sedative after-effects. Their food value depends largely on the amount of milk, cream and sugar put into them. Chocolate and cocoa are both drugs and foods. Alcohol is a stimulant at first, afterwards a sedative, and at all times an anesthetic.

When we think of drinking for the sake of supplying the bodily need of fluid, we should think of water and nothing else. If other liquids are taken, they should be taken as foods or drugs.

Water is the best solvent known. The alchemists of old spent much time and energy trying to find the universal solvent, believing that thereafter it would be easy to discover a method of making base metals noble. But they never found anything better than water. Water is the compound that in its various forms does most to change the earth upon which we live, and it is more necessary for the continuation of life than anything else except air.

Pure water does not exist in nature, that is, we have never found a compound of the composition H_2O. Water always contains other matter. The various salts are dissolved in it and it absorbs gases. The nearest we come to pure water is distilled. Pure water is an unsatisfied compound, and as soon as it is exposed it begins to absorb gases and take up salts and organic matter.

Pure water differs from clean water. Clean or potable water is a compound which contains a moderate amount of salts, but very little of organic matter. Bacteria should be practically absent. Water that contains much of nitrogenous substances is unfit to use.

If the water is very hard, heavily loaded with salts, it should not be used extensively as a drink, for if too much of earthy and mineral matter is taken into the system, the body is unable to get rid of all of them. The result is a tendency for deposits to form in the body. In places where the water is excessively charged with lime it has been noticed that the bones harden too early, which prevents full development of the body. If the bones of the skull are involved, it means that there will not be room enough for the brain. Such diseases are rare in this country, but in parts of Europe they are not uncommon. If the water is very hard, a good plan is to distill it and then add a little of the hard water to the distilled water.

People who partake of an excessive amount of various salts can perhaps drink distilled water to advantage, but those who take but a normal amount of the salts in their foods should have natural water.

Water forms three-fourths of the human body, more or less. It is needed in every process that goes on within the body. "To be dry is to die." Water keeps the various vital fluids in solution so that they can perform their function. Without water there would be no sense of taste, no digestion, no absorption of food, no excretion of debris, and hence no life. The water is the vehicle through which the nutritive elements are distributed to the billions of cells of the body, and it is also the vehicle which carries the waste to the various excretory organs.

We can live several weeks without food, but only a few days without water.

Hot water and ice-cold water are both irritants. Water may be taken either warm or cool. It is best to avoid the extremes.

The amount of water needed each twenty-four hours varies according to circumstances. Two quarts is a favorite prescription. Those who eat freely of succulent fruits and vegetables do not need as much as those who live more on dry foods. Salt in excess calls for an abnormal amount of water, for salt is a diuretic, robbing the tissues of their fluids and consequently more water has to be taken to keep up the equilibrium.

Naturally, more water is required when the weather is hot than when it is cool. On hot days warm water is more satisfying and quenches thirst more quickly than ice water. Warm water also stimulates kidney action, which is often sluggish in summer. Ice water is the least satisfactory of all, for the more one drinks the more he wants.

A normal body calls for what water it needs, and no more. An abnormal body is no guide for either the amount of food or drink necessary. Many people do not like the taste of water, especially in the morning. This means that the body is diseased. To a normal person cool water is always agreeable when it is needed, and it is needed in the morning. People with natural taste do not care for ice water, but other water is relished.

The common habit of drinking with meals is a mistake. Man is the only animal that does this, and he has to pay dearly for such errors. Taking a bite of food and washing it down with fluid lead to undermastication and overeating, and then the body suffers from autointoxication. A mouthful of food followed by a swallow of liquid forces the contents of the mouth into the stomach before the saliva has the opportunity to act.

The best way is to drink one or two glasses of water in the morning before breakfast. Partake of the breakfast, and all other meals, without taking any liquid. Sometimes there is a desire for a drink immediately after the meal is finished. If so, take some water slowly. If it is taken slowly a little will satisfy. If it is gulped down it may be necessary to take one or two glasses of water before being satisfied.

Those who have a tendency to drink too much during warm weather will find very slow drinking helpful in correcting it. If there is any digestive weakness, the liquid taken immediately after a meal should be warm and should not exceed a cupful. Those with robust digestion may take cool water.

Cold water chills the stomach. Digestion will not take place until the stomach has reached the temperature of about one hundred degrees Fahrenheit again, and if the stomach contents are chilled repeatedly the tendency is strong for the food to ferment pathologically, instead of being properly digested. For this reason it is not well to drink while there is anything left in the stomach to digest. As stomach digestion generally takes two or three hours at least, it is well to wait this long before taking water after finishing a meal, and then drink all that is desired until within thirty minutes of taking the next meal. If the thirst should become very insistent before two or three hours have elapsed since eating, take warm water. Those who eat food simply prepared and moderately seasoned are not troubled much with excessive thirst.

Two quarts of water daily should be sufficient for the adults under ordinary conditions. Here, as in eating, no exact amount will fit everybody. Make a habit of drinking at least a glass of water before breakfast, cleaning the teeth and rinsing the mouth before swallowing any, and then take what water the body asks for during the rest of the day. Taking too much water is not as injurious as overeating, but waterlogging the body has a weakening effect.

To drink with the meals is customary, not because it is necessary, but because we have a number of drinks which appeal to many people. Water is the drink par excellence.

A food-beverage that is used by many is cambric tea, which is made of hot water, one-third or one-fourth of milk and a little sweetening. Children generally like this on account of the sweetness. It may be taken with any meal, when fluid is needed, but the amount should be limited to a cupful. It is not well to dilute the digestive juices too much.

The water taken in the morning helps to start the body to cleanse itself. Water drinking is a great aid in overcoming constipation. Constipated people generally overeat. Less food and more water will prove helpful in overcoming the condition.

Unfortunately for the race, we have accustomed ourselves to partake of beverages containing injurious, poisonous substances. Inasmuch as this is the place to discuss the drugs contained in coffee and tea, I shall take the liberty of dwelling upon other habit-forming substances in the same chapter. They are all a part of the drug addictions of the race. For scientific discussion of these various substances I refer you to technical works. In this chapter will be found only a discussion of their relation to people's welfare, that is, to health and efficiency.

Coffee, tea and chocolate contain a poisonous alkaloid which is generally called caffeine. The theine in tea and the theobromine in cocoa are so similar to caffeine that chemists can not differentiate them. These drinks when first taken cause a gentle stimulation under which more work can be done than ordinarily, but this is followed by a reaction, and then the powers of body and mind wane so much that the average output of work is less than when the body is not stimulated. The temporary apparently beneficial effect is more than offset by the reaction and therefore partaking of these beverages makes people inefficient. Coffee is very hard on the nerves, causing irritation, which is always followed by premature physical degeneration.

Experiments of late indicate that children who use coffee do not come up to the physical and mental standard of those who abstain. The effect on the adults is not so marked because adults are more stable than children.

Those who are not used to coffee will be unable to sleep for several hours after partaking of a cup. Some people drink so much of it that they become accustomed to it.

Coffee is not generally looked upon as one of the habit-forming drugs, but it is. However, of all the drugs which create a craving in the system for a repetition of the dose, coffee makes the lightest fetters. It is surprising how often health-seekers inform the adviser that they "can not get along without coffee." If they would take a cup a few times a year, it would do no harm, but the daily use is harmful to all, even if they feel no bad effects and make it "very weak," which is a favorite statement of the women.

Smoking, drinking beer and drinking coffee have a tendency to overcome constipation in those who are not accustomed to these things, but their action can not be depended upon for any length of time and the cure is worse than the disease.

Tea drinking has much the same effect as coffee drinking, except that it is decidedly constipating. Perhaps this is because there is considerable of the astringent tannin in the tea leaves.

Chocolate is a valuable food. Those who eat of other aliments in moderation may partake of chocolate without harm, but if chocolate is used in addition to an excess of other food, the results are bad. The chocolate is so rich that it soon overburdens some of the organs of digestion, especially the liver. The Swiss consume much of this food and it is valuable in cases where it is necessary to carry concentrated rations.

Alcohol in some form seems to have been consumed by even very primitive people as far back as history goes. The Bible records an early case of intoxication from wine, and beer was brewed by the ancient Egyptians. So much has been consumed that some people have a subconscious craving for it. There are cases on record where the very first drink caused an uncontrollable demand for the drug. Fortunately these cases are very rare.

Alcohol is really not a stimulant, though it gives a feeling of glow, warmth and well-being at first, but this is followed by a great lowering of physical power, which gives rise to disagreeable sensations. Then the drinker needs more alcohol to stimulate him again. Then there is another depression with renewed demand: There is no end to the craving for the drug once it has mastered the individual. The lungs, heart, digestive organs, muscles, in fact, every structure in the body loses working capacity. Alcohol seems to have a special affinity for nervous tissue.

A glass of beer or wine taken daily is no more harmful than a cup of coffee per day, but the coffee drinker does not make of himself such a public nuisance and menace as the man often does who drinks alcohol to excess.

Formerly it was respectable to drink. Some of our most noted public men were drunkards. Now a drunkard could not maintain himself in a prominent public position very long. To drink like a gentleman was no disgrace. Now real gentlemen do not get drunk.

In backward Russia they are becoming alarmed about the inroads of vodka, and are trying to decrease its consumption. France is trying to teach total abstinence to its young men because it disqualifies so many of them from military service to drink. Scandinavia is temperance territory. The German Kaiser has recently given a warning against drinking. The United States discourages drinking in the army and navy. Field armies are not supplied with alcoholics. Drinking is becoming disreputable.

It is very difficult to prove the harm done by excessive drinking of tea and coffee, also by the use of much tobacco, even if we do know that it is so. Everyone knows something about the deleterious effect of alcohol upon the consumer. Solomon wrote: "Wine is a mocker, strong drink is raging, and whosoever is deceived thereby is not wise. Who hath wounds without cause? Who hath redness of eyes?"

Alcohol permanently impairs both body and mind. Depending on how much is taken, it may cause various ills, ranging from inflammation of the stomach to insanity. It reduces the power of the mind to concentrate and it diminishes the ability of the muscles to work. It reduces the resistance of the body and shortens life. Its first effect is to lull the higher faculties to sleep.

Most drunkards do not recover from their disease, for drunkenness is a disease. The various drugs given to cure the afflictions are delusions.

Strengthening the body, mind and the will and instilling higher ideals are the best methods of cure. Suggestive therapeutics, and the awakening of a strong resolve for a better life are powerful aids. Proper feeding should not be overlooked, for bad habits do not flourish in a healthy body.

Civilization necessitates self-control and considerable self-denial. Those who go in the line of least resistance are on the road to destruction. It is often necessary to overcome habits which produce temporary gratification of the senses.

According to Warden Tynan of the Colorado Penitentiary, 96 per cent. of the prisoners are brought there because they use alcohol. It is also well known that moral lapses are most common when the will is weakened through the use of liquor. Those who have the welfare of the race at heart are therefore compelled to give considerable thought to this subject. According to past experience, it will not help to try to legislate sobriety into the people. Education and industrialism are the factors which it seems to me will be most potent in solving the alcohol problem. Morality, which in the last analysis is a form of selfishness, will teach many that it is poor policy to reduce one's efficiency and thereby reduce the earning capacity and enjoyment of life.

More and more the employers of labor will realize that the use of alcohol decreases the reliability and worth of the worker. Many will take steps like the following:

"In formal recognition of the fact, established beyond dispute by the tests of the new psychology, that industrial efficiency decreases with indulgence in alcohol and is increased by abstinence from it, the managers of a manufacturing establishment in Chester, Penn., have attacked the temperance problem from a new angle.

"Unlike many railways and some other corporations, they do not forbid their employees to drink, but they offer 10 per cent. advance in wages to all who will take and keep--the teetotaler's pledge. Incidentally, a breaking of the promise will mean a permanent severance of relations, but there is no emphasizing of that point, it being confidently expected that the advantage of perfect sobriety will be as well realized on one side as on the other."

Business has during the past two centuries been the great civilizer, the great moral teacher. It has found that honesty and righteousness pay and that injustice is folly. Business has led the way to the acceptance of a new ethics, and new morals.

What has been said about alcohol applies to tobacco in a much smaller degree. The use of tobacco seems to lead to the use of alcohol. It retards the development of children. It is surely one of the causes of various diseases. Tobacco heart, sore throat and indigestion are well known to physicians.

Tobacco contains one of the deadliest of poisons known. One-sixteenth of a grain of nicotine may prove fatal. The reason there are so few deaths from acute tobacco poisoning is that but very little of the nicotine is absorbed.

Men who chew tobacco make themselves disagreeable to others. Smoking of cigarettes is to be condemned not only because it poisons the body, but causes inattention and inability to concentrate on the part of the smoker, as well. Every little while he feels the desire to take a smoke, and if smoking is forbidden he devises means of getting away. He robs his employer of time for which he is paid and injures himself.

The ability to work is decreased by indulgence in smoking. Recent experiments show that for a short time there is increased activity after a smoke, but the following depression is greater than the stimulation, so there is an actual loss.

A few years ago, according to Mr. Wilson, who was then Secretary of Agriculture, there were about 4,000,000 drug addicts or "dope fiends" in the United States. Without doubt this estimate was too high, for the proportion of addicts in the country is not as great as in the large cities. The drugs chiefly used are cocaine, opium, laudanum, morphine and heroin. These drugs are much more destructive than alcohol. Cocaine and heroin are the worst. It is very difficult to stop using any of them once the habit has been formed. Nearly every "fiend" dies directly or indirectly from the effect of his particular drug. Every one weakens the body so that there is not much resistance to offer to acute diseases. Every one destroys the will power so that a cure is exceedingly difficult.

It is well to bear in mind that all are not possessed of strong enough will power to resist their cravings and that some take to cocaine when they can not get liquor. Cocaine is far worse than alcohol.

People should be very careful about taking patent medicines. There is no excuse for taking them. The most popular ones have as their basis one of the habit-forming drugs.

Most of the soothing syrups contain opium in some form. To give babies opiates is a grave error, to speak mildly. It weakens the child, may lay the foundation for a deadly habit later in life, and often an overdose kills outright. Well informed mothers avoid such drugs and keep their children reasonably quiet by means of proper care.

Many of the remedies for nasal catarrh and hay fever contain much cocaine. Cocaine is an astringent and a painkiller and people mistake the temporary lessening of discharge from the nose and disappearance of pain for curative effects. But there is nothing curative about it. In a short time the mucous membrane relaxes again and then the discharge is re-established. The nerves which were put out of commission resume their function and then the pain reappears.

Opium or one of its derivatives is generally present in the patent medicines given for coughs. Opium is also an astringent and will suppress secretions, but this is not a cure. Excessive secretions are an indication that the body is surcharged with poison and food. Let them escape and then live so that there will be internal cleanliness and then there will be no more coughs and colds.

The unfortunate people who get into the habit of using these drugs degenerate physically, mentally and morally. They need more and more of their drug to produce the desired effect until they at last take enough daily to kill several normal men. Sometimes they are able to keep everybody in ignorance of what they are doing for years. They develop slyness and secretiveness. They become very suspicious. They are nearly always untruthful, and those who deal with them are surprised and wonder why those who used to be open and above-board now are furtive and dishonest. They often lie when there is not the slightest excuse for it. The moral disintegration is often the first sign noticed.

After habitually using any of these drugs for a while the body demands the continuation and if the victim is deprived of his accustomed portion there will be a collapse with intense suffering. Every tortured nerve in the body seems to call out for the drug. The victim will do anything to get his drug. He will lie, steal, and he may even attack those who are caring for him. For the time being he is insane.

Many professional men use cocaine. It is a favorite with writers. It often shows in their work. Those who write under the inspiration of this drug often do some good work, but they are unable to keep to their subject. Their writings lack order. We have enough of such writings to have them classified as "cocaine literature."

If there are 4,000,000, or even fewer, of these people in our land, it is a serious problem, for every one is a degenerate, to a certain degree. If the medical profession and the druggists would co-operate it would be easy enough to prevent the growth of a new crop of dope fiends. Of course, people would have to stop taking patent medicines, which often start the victims on the road to degeneration. Then the physicians should stop prescribing habit-forming drugs, as well as all other drugs, and teach the people that physical, mental and moral salvation come through right living and right thinking.

Unfortunately the medical profession is careless and is responsible for the existence of many of the drug addicts. A patient has a severe pain. What is the easiest way to satisfy him? To give a hypodermic injection of some opiate. The patient, not realizing the danger, demands a pain-killer every time he suffers. He soon learns what he is getting and then he goes to the drug store and outfits himself with a hypodermic outfit and drugs, and the first thing he knows he is a slave, in bondage for life. This is no exaggeration. There are hundreds of thousands of victims to the drug habit who trace their downfall to the treatment received at the hands of reputable physicians, who do not look upon their practice with the horror it should inspire because it is so common. Doctors do not always bury their mistakes. Some of them walk about for years.

In spite of laws against the sale of various drugs, they can be obtained.

There are doctors and druggists of easy conscience who are very accommodating, for a price.

There is no legitimate need for the use of one-hundredth of the amount of these drugs that is now consumed. A local injection of cocaine for a minor operation is justifiable, but none of the habit-forming drugs should be used in ordinary practice to kill pain, for the proper application of water in conjunction with right living will do it better and there are no evil after effects. Massage is often sufficient.

To show a little more clearly how some people become addicted to drugs, let us consider one of the latest, heroin: A few years ago this drug, which is an opium derivative, was practically unknown. It is much stronger than morphine and consequently the effect can be obtained more quickly by means of a smaller dose. Physicians thought at first that it was not a habit-forming drug, for they could use it over a longer period of time than they could employ morphine, without establishing the craving and the habit. So they began to prescribe heroin instead of morphine, and many a morphine addict was advised to substitute heroin. All went well for a short while, until the victims found that they were enslaved by a drug that was even worse than morphine. Now, thanks chiefly to the medical profession, it is estimated that we have in our land several hundred thousand heroin addicts. Sallow of face, gaunt of figure, looking upon the world through pin-point pupils, with all of life's beauty, hope and joy gone, they are marching to premature death.

The medical profession furnishes more than its proportion of drug addicts. They know the danger of the drugs, but familiarity breeds contempt. If the public but knew how many of their medical advisers, who should always be clear-minded, are befuddled by drugs, there would be a great awakening. One eminent physician who has now been in practice about forty-five years and has had much experience with drug addicts, has said that according to his observations, about one physician in four contracts the drug habit. I believe this is exaggerated, but I am acquainted with a number of physicians who are addicts.

Physicians who smoke do not condemn the practice. Those who drink are likely to prescribe beer and wine for their patients. Those who are addicted to drugs use them too liberally in their practice.

Those who have watched the effects of the various drugs, from coffee to heroin, must condemn their use. It is true that an occasional cup of coffee or tea, a glass of wine or beer does no harm. A cigarette a week would not hurt a boy, nor would on occasional cigar harm a man. But how many people are willing to indulge occasionally? The rule is that they indulge not only daily, but several times a day, and the results are bad. One bad habit leads to another, and the time always comes when it is a choice between disease and early death on one hand, and the giving up of the bad habits on the other, and when this time comes the bonds of habits are often so strong that the victim is unable to break them.

I realize that knowledge will not always keep people out of temptation and that some individuals will take the broad way that leads to destruction in spite of anything that may be said. Youth is impatient of restraint and ever anxious for new experiences. Regarding this serious matter of destructive drug use, much could be done by teaching people their place in society: That is, what they owe to themselves, their families and the public in general. In other words, teach the young people the higher selfishness, part of which consists of considerable self-control, self-denial and self-respect.

Drugs are too easy to obtain today. Some day people will be so enlightened that they will not allow themselves to be medicated. This is the trend of the times. Until such a time comes, society should protect itself by making it very difficult to get any of the habit-forming drugs. If necessary, the free hand of the physician should be stayed. Much of the confidence blindly given him is misplaced.

CHAPTER XXI.

CARE OF THE SKIN.

The skin is neglected and abused. Very few realize how important it is to give this organ the necessary attention. If we were living today as our ancestors doubtless lived, we could neglect the skin, as they did. They wore little or no clothing. The skin, which formerly was very hairy, served as protection. It was exposed to the elements, which toughened it and kept it active.

Today most people give the skin too great protection, and thus weaken it. The result is that it degenerates and partly loses its function with consequent detriment to the individual's health.

A normal skin has a very soft feel, imparting to the fingers a pleasant, vital sensation. It either has color or suggests color. An abnormal skin pleases neither the sense of seeing nor feeling. It may feel inert or it may be inflamed.

The skin is a beautiful and complex structure. It is made up of an outer layer called the epidermis and an inner layer, the true skin or corium, which rests upon a subcutaneous layer, composed principally of fat and connective tissue.

The epidermis is divided into four layers. It has no blood-vessels and no nerves, but is nourished by lymph which escapes from the vessels deeper in the skin. It is simply protective in nature.

The true skin is made up of two indistinct layers, which harbor a vast multitude of nerves, blood-vessels and lymph-vessels.

In the skin there are two kinds of glands, the sebaceous and the sweat glands. The sebaceous glands are, as a general rule, to be found in greatest numbers on the hairiest parts of the body and are absent from the palms of the hands and the soles of the feet. They throw off a secretion known as sebum, which is made up principally of dead cells that have undergone fatty degeneration and of other debris. The sebum serves as lubricant. It is generally discharged near or at the shaft of a hair.

The sweat glands discharge on the average from one and one-half to two pounds of perspiration per day, more in hot weather and much less when it is cool. They are distributed over the whole external surface of the body. According to Krause there are almost 2,400,000 of them. They carry off water and carbonic acid gas chiefly.

The functions of the skin are: To protect the underlying structures; to regulate the heat; to serve as an organ of respiration; to serve as an organ of touch and thermal sensation; to secrete and eliminate various substances from the body; to absorb.

The heat regulation is quite automatic. When the external temperature is high there is a relaxation of the skin. The pores open, the perspiration goes to the surface and evaporates, thus cooling the body. When the surface is cool the skin contracts, closing the pores and conserving the heat. Radiation always takes place, except when the temperature is very high.

The sensation of touch and the ability to feel heat and cold protect us from untold numbers of dangers. They are a part of the equipment which enables us to adjust our selves to our environment.

The secretions and excretions are perspiration and sebum. These contain water, carbonic acid, urea, buturic acid, formic acid, acetic acid, salts, the chief being sodium chloride, and many other substances.

The respiratory function consists in the absorption of a small amount of oxygen and the giving off of some carbonic acid.

A small amount of water can be absorbed by the skin. Oils can also be absorbed. In case of malnutrition in children, olive-oil rubs are often helpful. This absorptive function is taken advantage of by physicians who rub various medicaments into the skin. Mercury enough to produce salivation can be absorbed in this way.

From the above it will be seen that the skin is not only complex in structure, but has many functions. It is impossible to have perfect health without a good skin. Under civilized conditions a healthy skin can not be had without giving it some care. The average person has a skin that shows lack of care. Fortunately, but little care is needed.

A bath should be taken often enough to ensure cleanliness. Warm water and soap need not be used more than once or twice a week under ordinary conditions. If the soap causes itching, it is well to use a small amount of olive oil on the body afterwards, rubbing it in thoroughly, and going over the body with a soft cloth after the oil rub, thus removing the oil which would otherwise soil the clothes. If the skin is not kept clean, the millions of pores are liable to be partly stopped up, which results in the retention of a part of the excretory matter within the skin, where it may cause enough irritation to produce some form of cutaneous disorder, or the skin may through disuse become so inactive that too much work is thrown upon the other excretory organs, which may also become diseased from overwork and excessive irritation.

Soaps are irritants. Tallow soaps and olive oil soaps are less irritating than other varieties. Whatever kind of soap is used, it should be rinsed off thoroughly, for if some of it is left in the pores of the skin roughness or even mild inflammation may ensue. Be especially careful about the soap used for babies, avoiding all highly colored and cheap perfumed soaps.

Whether to take a daily sponge bath or not is a matter of no great importance, and each individual can safely suit himself. If there is quick reaction and a feeling of warmth and well-being following a cold sponge, it is all right. If the skin remains blue and refuses to react for a long time, the cold sponge bath is harmful. The cold plunge is always a shock, and no matter how strong a person may be, frequent repetition is not to be recommended. People who take cold plunges say that they do no harm, but it is well to remember that life is not merely a matter of today and tomorrow, but of next year, or perhaps forty, fifty or sixty years from today. A daily shock may cause heart disease in the course of twenty or thirty years.

A good way to take a cold bath is to get under a warm shower and gradually turn off the warm water. Then stand under the cold shower long enough to rinse well the entire surface of the body.

Those who take cold sponge baths in winter and find them severe, should precede the sponging in cold water with a quick sponging off with tepid water, and they should always take these baths in a warm room.

After all baths give the body a good dry rubbing, using brisk movements. Bath towels, flesh brushes or the open hands may be used for the dry rubbing.

The sponge bath has practically no value as a cleanser. Its chief virtue consists in stimulating the circulation of the blood and the lymph in the skin. In summer it is cooling. It is important to have good surface circulation, but this can be attained as well by means of dry rubbing. The rubbing is more important than wetting the skin. A skin that is rubbed enough becomes so active that it practically cleans itself, and it protects against colds and other diseases. Some advocate dispensing with the bath entirely, but that is going to extremes. Cleanliness is worth while for the self-respect it gives the individual.

Hot baths are weakening and relaxing, hence weak people should not stay long in the hot bath. Cold baths are stimulating to strong people and depressing to those who do not react well from them. Swimming is far different from taking a cold bath. A person who can swim with benefit and comfort for twenty minutes would have a chill, perhaps, if he remained for five minutes in the bath tub in water of the same temperature. Swimming is such an active exercise that it aids the circulation, keeping the blood pretty well to the surface in spite of the chilling effect of the water.

If a very warm bath is taken, there should be plenty of fresh air in the bath room and it is well to sip cold water while in the bath and keep a cloth wrung out of cold water on the forehead. People who are threatened with a severe cold or pneumonia can give themselves no better treatment than to take a hot bath, as hot as they can stand it, lasting for one-half hour to an hour, drinking as much warm water as can be taken with comfort both before and after getting into the tub. This bath must be taken in very warm water, otherwise it will do no good. It is weakening and relaxing, but through its relaxing influence it equalizes the circulation of the blood, bringing much to the surface that was crowding the lungs and other internal organs, thus causing the dangerous congestion that so often ends in pneumonia. After the bath wrap up well so that the perspiration will continue for some time. When the sweating is over, get into dry clothes and remain in bed for six to eight hours. To make assurance doubly sure, give the bowels a good cleaning out with either enemas or cathartics, or both. Then eat nothing until you are comfortable. Such treatment would prevent much pneumonia and many deaths. The best preventive is to live so that sudden chilling does not produce pneumonia or other diseases, which it will not do in good health.

People with serious diseases of the heart, arteries or of the kidneys should not take protracted or severe baths.

To sum up the use of water on the skin: Use enough to be clean. No more is necessary. The application of water should be followed by thorough drying and dry rubbing. If the reaction is poor, do not remain in cold water long enough to produce chilling. As a rule thin people should use but little cold water, and they should never remain long in cold water.

Water intelligently applied to the skin in disease is a splendid aid in cleansing the system. It is surprising what a great amount of impurity can be drawn from the body by means of wet packs. However, this is a treatise on health, so we shall not go into details here regarding hydrotherapy.

No matter what one's ideas may be on the subject of bathing, there can hardly be more than one opinion regarding the application of dry friction to the skin. Those who have noted its excellent results feel that it should be a daily routine. It should be practiced either morning or evening, or both. From five to ten minutes spent thus daily will pay high dividends in health. A vigorous rubbing is exercise not only for the skin, but for nearly every muscle in the body.

The dry rubbing keeps the surface circulation vigorous. The surface circulation, and especially the circulation in the hands and the feet, is the first part that begins to stagnate. Blood stagnation means the beginning of the process which results in old age. In other words, dry friction to the skin helps to preserve health and youth. Skin that is not exercised often becomes very hard and scales off particles of mineral matter.

If women would put less dependence on artificial beautifiers and more on scientific massage, they would get much better results. They would avoid many a wrinkle and save their complexions. The neck and the face should never be massaged downwards. The strokes should be either upwards or from side to side, the side strokes generally being toward the median line. Such massaging will prevent the sagging of the face muscles for years and help to keep the face free from wrinkles and young in appearance. The massaging should be rather gentle, for if it is too vigorous the tendency is to remove the normal amount of fat that pads and rounds out the face. Men can do the same thing, but most men have no objection to wrinkles.

However, most men do object to baldness, which can be prevented in nearly every case. To produce hair on a polished pate is a different proposition. It is indeed difficult. If you will look at a picture of the circulation of the blood in the scalp, you will notice that the arteries supplying it come from above the eye sockets in front, from before and behind the ears on the sides, and from the nape of the neck in the rear. They spread out and become smaller and smaller as they travel toward the top of the head, and especially toward the back. The scalp is well supplied with blood, but it is not given much exercise. The tendency is for the blood stream to become sluggish, deposits gradually forming in the walls of the blood-vessels, which make them less elastic and decrease the size of the lumen. The result is less food for the hair roots and food of inferior quality.

This process of cutting off the circulation in the scalp is largely aided by the tight hats and caps worn by men, which compress the blood-vessels. It is quite noticeable that people with round heads have a greater tendency to become bald than those with more irregular heads. The reason is probably that the hats fit more snugly on the round-headed people. There are many exceptions. Women are not so prone to baldness as men, because they wear hats that do not exclude the air from the hair nor do they compress the blood-vessels.

Let those men who dislike to lose their hair massage the scalp for a short while daily, beginning above the eyes, in front of the ears and at the nape of the neck and going to the top of the head. Then let them wear as sensible hats as possible, avoiding those that exert great pressure on the blood-vessels that feed the scalp. Thus they will not only be able to retain their hair much longer than otherwise, but the hair that is well fed does not fade as early as that which lives on half rations.

In the case of preserving the hair, an ounce of prevention is worth a ton of cure. The man who can produce a satisfactory hair restorer that will give results without any effort on the part of the men can become a millionaire in a short time.

The hair is a modified form of skin. Each hair is supplied with blood, and the reason that the hair stands up during intense fear is that to the lower part of the shaft is attached a little muscle. During fear this contracts, as do other involuntary muscles, and then the hair stands up straight instead of being oblique.

As a rule people protect the skin too much. The best protection they have against cold is a good circulation. With a poor circulation it is difficult to keep warm in spite of much clothing. Coldness is also largely a state of mind. People get the idea of cold into the head and then it is almost impossible for them to keep warm. On the same winter day we may see a man in a thick overcoat trying to shrink into himself, shivering, while a lady passes blithely by, with her bosom bared to the wind.

The face tolerates the cold, because it is used to it, the neck and the upper part of the chest likewise, and so it would be with the skin of the entire body if we accustomed it to be exposed. We use too heavy clothes. It is a mistake to hump the back and draw in the shoulders during cold weather, for this reduces the lung capacity, thus depriving the body of its proper amount of oxygen. The result is that there is not enough combustion to produce the necessary amount of heat.

Wool is warm covering, the best we have. However, it is very irritating to the skin and has a tendency to make the wearer too warm. It does not dry out readily. Consequently the wearer remains damp a long time after perspiring. The result is a moist, clammy skin. A skin thus pampered in damp warmth becomes delicate, and like other hot-house products unable to hold its own when exposed to inclement weather. A good way to take cold easily is to wear wool next to the skin. The best recipe for getting cold feet is to wear woolen stockings. Wear cotton or linen or silk next to the skin. Cotton is satisfactory and cheap. Linen is excellent, but a good suit of linen underwear is too costly for the average purse. Remie, said to be the linen of the Bible, is highly recommended by some.

Those working indoors should wear the same kind of underwear summer and winter, and it should be very light. If people use heavy underwear in heated rooms, they become too warm. The consequence is that when they go out doors they are chilled, and if they are not in good physical condition colds and other diseases generally result. By wearing outer garments according to climatic conditions one can easily get all the protection necessary. Those who take the proper food and enough exercise and dry friction of the skin will not require or desire an excessive amount of clothing. The feel of the wintry blast on the skin is not disagreeable.

If we would only give the skin more exercise, through rubbing, and more fresh air, we would soon discard much of our clothing, and wear but enough to make a proper and modest appearance in public, with extra covering on cold days. Nothing can be much more ridiculous and uncomfortable than a man in conventional attire on a hot summer's day.

Of course, thin, nervous people should not expose themselves too much to the cold.

Most of the diseases known by the name of skin diseases, are digestive troubles and blood disorders manifesting in the skin. As soon as the systemic disease upon which they depend disappears, these so-called skin diseases get well. Erysipelas is one of the so-called germ diseases, but it is controlled very quickly by a proper diet. It can not occur in people until they have ruined their health by improper living. Pure blood will not allow the development of the streptococcus erysipelatis in sufficient numbers to cause trouble. First the disease develops and then the germ comes along and multiplies in great numbers, giving it type.

Acne, which is very common for a few years after puberty, shows a bad condition of the blood. Even during the changes that occur at puberty no disease will manifest in healthy boys and girls. About this time the young people eat excessively, the result being indigestion and impure blood. The changes that occur in the skin make it a favorable place for irritations to manifest. Let the boys and girls eat so that they have bright eyes and clean tongues and there will be very little trouble from disfiguring pimples.

Eczema is generally curable by means of proper diet and the same is true of nearly all skin diseases that afflict infants.

There are diseases of the skin due to local irritants, such as the various forms of trade eczema, scabies (itch), and pediculosis (lousiness), but the fact remains that nearly all skin diseases fail to develop if the individual eats properly, and most of them can be cured, after they have developed, by proper diet and attention to hygiene generally. If the diet is such that irritants are manufactured in the alimentary tract and absorbed into the blood, and then excreted through the skin, where enough irritation is produced to cause disease, it is useless to treat with powders and salves.

Correct the dietetic errors and the skin will cure itself. Specialists in skin diseases often fail because they treat this organ as an independent entity, instead of considering it as a part of the body whose health depends mostly upon the general health.

CHAPTER XXII.

EXERCISE.

Nature demands of us that we use our mental and physical powers in order to get the best results. Man was made to be active. In former times he had to earn his bread in the sweat of his face or starve. Now we have evolved, or is it a partial degeneration, into a state where a sharp mind commands much more of the means of sustenance than does physical exertion. The consequence is that many of those equipped with the keenest minds fail to keep their bodies active. This helps to lessen their resistance and produces early death.

Some exercise is needed and the question is, how much is necessary and how is it to be taken so that it will not degenerate into drudgery? There are very few with enough persistence to continue certain exercises, no matter how beneficial, if they become a grind.

The amount required depends upon the circumstances. Ordinarily, a few minutes of exercise each day, supplemented with some walking and deep breathing will suffice. About five minutes of vigorous exercise night and morning are generally enough to keep a person in good physical condition, if he is prudent otherwise.

Many strive to build up a great musculature. This is a mistake, unless the intention is to become an exhibit for the sake of earning one's living. Big muscles do not spell health, efficiency and endurance. Even a dyspeptic may be able to build big muscles. What is needed for the work of life is not a burst of strength that lasts for a few moments and then leaves the individual exhausted for the day, but the endurance which enables one to forge ahead day after day.

It is generally dangerous to build up great muscles, for if the exercises that brought them into being are stopped, they begin to degenerate so fast that the system with difficulty gets rid of the poisons. Then look out for one of the diseases of degeneration, such as inflammation of the kidneys or typhoid fever.

The great muscles exhibited from time to time upon the variety stage and in circuses are not normal. Man is the only animal that develops them, and they are not brought about by ordinary circumstances. Once acquired, they prove a burden, for they demand much daily work to be kept in condition.

Good muscles are more serviceable than extraordinary ones. Vigorous exercise is better than violent exercise. It is well known that many of our picked athletes, men with great original physical endowment, die young. The reason is that they have either been overdeveloped, or at some time they have overtaxed their bodies so in a supreme effort at vanquishing their opponents that a part of the vital mechanism has been seriously affected. Then when they settle down to business life they fail to take good care of themselves and they degenerate rapidly.

Exercising should not be a task, for then it is work. It should be of a kind that interests and pleases the individual, for then it is accompanied by that agreeable mental state from which great good will come to the body. It is necessary for us to think enough of our bodies to supply them with the activity needed for their welfare and we should do this with good grace.

Exercise enough to bring the various muscles into play and the heart into vigorous action. Office workers should take exercises for the part of the body above the waist, plus some walking each day. All should take enough exercise to keep the spine straight and pliable. Bending exercises are good for this purpose, keeping the knees straight and touching the floor with the fingers. Then bend backward as far as possible. Then with hands on the hips rotate the body from the waist.

It is very desirable to keep the body erect, for this gives the greatest amount of lung space, and gives the individual a noble, courageous appearance and feeling. The forward slouch is the position of the ape. It is not necessary to pay any attention to the shoulders, if the spine is kept in proper position, for the shoulders will then fall into the right place. Being straight is a matter of habit. No one can maintain this position without some effort. At least, one has to make the effort to get and retain the habit. Most round-shouldered people could school themselves in two or three months to be straight.

Those who are moderate in eating need less exercise than others. Too great food intake requires much labor to work it off. When the food is but enough to supply materials for repair, heat and energy, there is no need of great effort to burn up the excess. To exercise much and long, then eat enough to compel more exercise, is a waste of good food, time and energy. Be moderate in all things if you would have the best that life can give you.

Always make deep breathing a part of the exercise. No matter what one's physical troubles may be, deep breathing will help to overcome them. It will help to cure cold feet by bringing more oxygen into the blood. It will help to drive away constipation by giving internal massage to the bowels. It will help to overcome torpid liver by the exercise given that organ. It will help to cure rheumatism by producing enough oxygen to burn up some of the foreign deposits in various parts of the body. As an eye-opener deep breathing has alcohol distanced. It costs nothing and has only good after effects. Moreover, deep breathing takes no time. A dozen or more deep breaths can be taken morning and night, and every time one steps into the fresh air, without taking one second from one's working time. To have health good blood is necessary, and this can not be had without taking sufficient fresh air into the lungs.

Proper clothing must also be taken into consideration in connection with breathing and exercise. The clothes must be loose enough to allow free play to limbs, chest and abdomen. Men and women were not shaped to wear two and three inch heels. Those who persist in this folly must pay the price in discomfort and an unbalanced body.

The time to take exercise depends upon circumstances. It is best not to indulge for at least one or two hours after a hearty meal, for exercise interferes with digestion. A very good plan is to take from five to twenty-five minutes of exercise, according to one's requirement, before dressing in the morning and after undressing at night. Those who take exercises in a gymnasium or have time for out door games will have no difficulty in selecting proper time.

Dumbbells, Indian clubs, weights, patent exercisers and gymnasium stunts are all right for those who enjoy them. One thing to bear in mind is that short, choppy movements are not as good as the larger movements that bring the big muscles into play.

It is well to exercise until there is a comfortable feeling of fatigue. If this is done the heart works vigorously, sending the blood rapidly to all parts of the body, and the lungs also come into full play to supply the needed oxygen. This acts as a tonic to the entire system.

The body must be used to keep it from degenerating. A healthy body gives courage and an optimistic outlook upon life. A sluggish liver can hide the most beautiful sunrise, but a healthy body gives the eye power to see beauty on the most dreary day.

Those who are not accustomed to exercise will be very, sore at first, if they begin too vigorously. The soreness can be avoided by taking but two or three minutes at a time at first, and increasing until the desired amount is taken daily.

If the muscles get a little sore and stiff at first, do not quit, for by continuing the exercises, the soreness soon leaves. Many begin with great enthusiasm, which soon burns itself out. Excessive enthusiasm is like the burning love of those who "can't live" without the object of their affection. It burns so brightly that it soon consumes itself. Go to work at a rate that can be kept up. To exercise hard for a few weeks or a few months and then give it up will do no good in the end. However, a person may occasionally let a day or two pass by without taking exercise with benefit. Avoid getting into a monotonous grind.

I believe that the very best exercises are those which are taken in the spirit of play. No matter who it is, if he or she will make the effort, time enough can be found occasionally to spend at least one-half of a day in the open, and this is very important. We can not long flourish without getting into touch with mother nature, and we need a few hours each week without care and worry in her company. Many immediately say, "I can't." Get rid of that negative attitude and say, "I can and I will." See how quickly the obstacles melt away.

There are many who are slaves to duty. They believe that they must grind away. They think they are indispensable. The world got along very well before they were born and it will roll on in the same old way after they are gathered to their fathers. The thing to do is to break the bonds of the wrong mental attitude and then both time and opportunity will be forthcoming.

I shall comment on only a few of the outdoor exercises that are excellent.

Swimming is one of the finest. There is a great deal of difference between swimming and taking a bath in a tub. Some people cannot remain in the water long, but if they have any resistance at all and are active, there will be no bad results. In swimming it is well to take various strokes, swimming on the back, on the side, and on the face. This brings nearly every muscle in the body into play and if the swimmer does not stay in too long it makes him feel fine. If a feeling of chilliness or weariness is experienced, it is time to quit the water, dry off well and take a vigorous dry rub. Swims should always be followed with considerable rubbing. The use of a little olive oil on the body, and especially on the feet, is very grateful. No special rule can be laid down for the duration of a swim, but very thin people should generally not remain in the water more than fifteen minutes, and stout, vigorous ones not over an hour. It is best not to go swimming until two hours have elapsed since the last meal.

Every boy and every girl should be taught to swim, for it may be the means of preserving their lives. It is not difficult. For the benefit of those who start the beginners with the rather tedious and tiresome breast stroke, will say that the easiest way to teach swimming is to get the learner to float on his back. I have taught boys to float in as little as three minutes, and after that everything else is easy. When the beginner can float, he can easily start to paddle a little and make some progress. Then he can turn on his side and learn the side stroke, which is one of the best. Then he can turn on the face and learn various strokes. This is not the approved way of learning to swim, but it is the easiest and quickest way.

To float simply means to get into balance in the water. It is necessary to arch the body, making the spine concave posteriorly, and bending the neck well backward at first. In the beginning it is a great aid to fill the lungs well and breathe rather shallow. This makes the body light in the water. Tell the beginner that it does not make any difference whether the feet sink or stay up. It is only necessary to keep the face above water while floating. If there is the slightest tendency to sink, bend the neck a little more, putting the head, farther back in the water, instead of raising it, as most of the learners want to do. Remember that the trunk and neck must be kept well arched, the head well back in the water. The moment the beginner doubles up at waist or hips or bends the neck forward, raising the head, he sinks.

For speed and fancy swimming professional instruction should be obtained. Swimming is one of the best all-round developers, as well as one of the most pleasant of exercises.

Golf is no longer a rich man's game. The large cities have public links. For an office man it is a splendid game. Women can play it with equal benefit. The full vigorous strokes, followed with a walk after the ball, then more strokes, exercise the entire body. It is good for young and old, and for people in all walks of life.

Tennis is splendid for some people. Those who are very nervous and excitable should play at something else, for they are apt to play too hard and use up too much energy. Overexercising is just as harmful as excesses in other lines. Tennis requires quickness and is a good game for those who are inclined to be sluggish, for it wakes them up.

Horseback riding is also a fine exercise. The companionship with an intelligent animal, the freedom, the fresh air, the scenery, all give enjoyment of life, and the constant movement acts as a most delicious tonic. There is only one correct way to ride for both sexes, and that is astride. The side saddle position keeps the spine twisted so that it takes away much of the benefit to be derived from riding. Out west the approved manner of riding for women is astride. The women of the west make a fine appearance on horseback.

Tramping is possible for all. If there are hills to be climbed, or mountains, so much the better. Put on old clothes and old shoes and have an enjoyable time. Fine apparel under the circumstances spoils more than half of the pleasure.

Playing ball or bicycle riding may be indulged in with benefit. It is not fashionable to ride on bicycles today, yet it is a pleasant mode of covering ground, and if the trunk is kept erect it is a good exercise. Jumping rope, playing handball, tossing the medicine ball and sawing wood are good forms of exercise and great fun. The spirit of play and good will easily double the value of any exercise that is taken.

Dancing is also good if the ventilation is adequate and the hours are reasonable.

Under various conditions vicarious exercises are valuable, and by that I mean such forms of exercise as massage, osteopathic treatment or vibratory treatment. If anything is wrong with the spine, get an osteopath or a chiropractor. They can help to remedy such defects more quickly than anyone else. They are experts in adjustments and thrusts.

Some people take exercises while lying in bed or on the floor. One good exercise to take while lying on the back is to go through the motions of riding a bicycle. Another is to lie down, then bend the body at the hips, getting into a sitting position; repeat a few times. Another is to face the floor, holding the body rigid, supported on the toes and the palms of the hands; slowly raise the body until the arms are straight and slowly lower it again until the abdomen touches the floor; repeat several times.

It is impossible to go into detail regarding various exercises here. Those who wish to take care of themselves can easily devise a number of good ones, or they can employ a physical culture teacher to give them pointers. Here as elsewhere, good sense wins out. It is not necessary to give much time to exercise, but a little is valuable. Those who labor with their hands often use but few muscles, and it would be well for them to take corrective exercises so that the body will remain in good condition.

There is no excuse for round shoulders and sunken chests. A few weeks, or at most a few months, will correct this in young people. The older the individual, the longer it takes. If the vertebrae have grown together in bony union no correction is possible.

It is as necessary to relax as it is to exercise. When weary, take a few minutes off and let go physically and mentally. A little training will enable you to drop everything, and even if it is for but five minutes, the ease gives renewed vigor. It does not matter what position is assumed, if it is comfortable and allows the muscles to lose all tension. At such times it is well to let the eyelids gently close, giving the eyes a rest. Eye strain is very exhausting to the whole body and often results in serious discomfort.

Many do not know how to relax. They think they are relaxed, yet their bodies are in a state of tension. When relaxed any part of the body that may be raised falls down again as though it were dead. People who do much mental work are at times so aroused by ideas that refuse to release their hold until they have been worked out or given expression that they can not sleep for the time being. A few minutes of relaxation then gives rest. When the problem has been solved, the worker is rewarded with sweet slumbers. An occasional night of this kind of wakefulness does no harm, provided no such drugs as coffee, alcohol, strychnine and morphine are used.

We are undoubtedly intended to be useful. Normal men and women are not content unless they are helpful. Hence we have our work or vocation. However, people who get into a rut, and they are liable to if they work all the time at one thing, lose efficiency. Therefore it is well to have an avocation or a hobby to sharpen mind and body.

It does not make much difference what the hobby is, provided it is interesting. We waste much time that could give us more pleasure if it were intelligently employed. An hour a day given to a subject for a few years in the spirit of play will give a vast fund of information and may in time be of inestimable benefit.

Those who labor much with the hands would do well to take some time each day for mental recreation, and those who work in mental channels should get joy and benefit from physical efforts. A few hobbies, depending upon circumstances, may be: Photography, music, a foreign language, the drama, literature, history, philosophy, painting, gardening, raising chickens, dogs or bees, floriculture, and botany. Some people have become famous through their hobbies. They are excellent for keeping the mind fluid, which helps to retain physical youth.

There is something peculiarly beneficial about tending and watching growing and unfolding things. It is well known that women remain young longer than men. We have good reason to believe that one of the causes is their intimate relation with children. Growing flowers, vegetables, chickens and pups have the same influence in lesser degree. Tender, helpless things bring out the best qualities in our natures. We can not be on too intimate terms with nature, so, if possible, select a hobby that brings you closely in contact with her and her products.

CHAPTER XXIII.

BREATHING AND VENTILATION.

The respiratory apparatus is truly marvelous in beauty and efficiency. Medical men complain about nature's way of constructing the alimentary canal, saying that it is partly superfluous, but no such complaint is lodged against the lungs and their accessories.

The respiratory system may be likened in form to a well branched tree, with hollow trunk, limbs and leaves: The trachea is the trunk; the two bronchi, one going to the right side and the other to the left side, are the main branches; the bronchioles and their subdivisions are the smaller branches and twigs; the air cells are the leaves.

The trachea and bronchi are tubes, furnished with cartilaginous rings to keep them from collapsing. They are lined with mucous membrane. The bronchi give off branches, which in turn divide and subdivide, until they become very fine. Upon the last subdivisions are clustered many cells or vesicles. These are the air cells and here the exchange takes place, the blood giving up carbonic acid gas and receiving from the inspired air a supply of oxygen. This exchange takes place through a very thin layer of mucous membrane, the air being on one side and the blood capillaries on the other side.

The whole respiratory tract is lined with mucous membrane. This membrane is ciliated, that is, it is studded with tiny hairlike projections, extending into the air passages. These are constantly in motion, much like the grain in a field when the wind is gently blowing. Their function is to prevent the entry of foreign particles into the air cells, for their propulsive motion is away from the lungs, toward the external air passages.

In some of the large cities where the atmospheric conditions are unfavorable and the air is laden with dust and smoke, the cilia are unable to prevent the entrance of all the fine foreign particles in the air. Then these particles irritate the mucous membrane, which secretes enough mucus to imprison the intruders. Consequently there is occasionally expulsion of gray or black mucus, which should alarm no one under the circumstances, if feeling well. Normally the mucous membrane secretes only enough mucus to lubricate itself, and when there is much expulsion of mucus it means that either the respiratory or the digestive system, or both, are being abused. At such times the sufferer should take an inventory of his habits and correct them.

The air cells are made up of very thin membrane. So great is their surface that if they could be flattened out they would form a sheet of about 2,000 square feet. We can not explain satisfactorily why it is that through their walls there is an exchange of gases, nor how the respiratory system can act so effectively both as an exhaust of harmful matter and a supply of necessary elements. The distribution of the blood capillaries, so tiny that the naked eye can not make them out, is wonderful. Under the microscope they look like patterns of delicate, complex, beautiful lace.

The lungs are supplied with more blood than any other, part of the body. A small part of it is for the nourishment of the lung structure, but most of it comes to be purified. After the blood has traveled to various parts of the body to perform its work as a carrier of food, and oxygen and gatherer of waste, it returns to the heart and from the heart it is sent to the lungs. There it gives up its carbonic acid gas and receives a supply of oxygen. Then it returns to the heart again and once more it is sent to all parts of the body to distribute the vital element, oxygen.

The lungs give off watery vapor, a little animal matter and considerable heat, but their chief function is to exchange the carbonic acid gas of the blood for the oxygen of the air. When the fats, sugars and starches, in their modified form, are burned in the body to produce heat and energy, carbonic acid gas and water are formed. The gas is taken up by the blood stream, which is being deprived of its oxygen at the same time. This exchange turns the blood from red into a bluish tinge. The red color is due to the union of oxygen with the iron in the blood corpuscles, forming rust, roughly speaking.

The fine adjustment that exists in nature can be seen by taking into consideration that animals give off carbon dioxide and breathe in oxygen, while vegetation exhales oxygen and inhales carbon dioxide. In other words, animal life makes conditions favorable for plant growth, and vegetation makes possible the existence of animals.

An animal of the higher class can live several days without water, several weeks without food, but only a very few minutes without oxygen. When the blood becomes surcharged with carbonic acid gas, and oxygen is refused admittance to the lungs, life ceases in about five or six minutes. From this it can easily be seen how important it is to have a proper supply of oxygen. Acute deprivation of this element is immediately fatal, and chronic deprivation of a good supply helps to produce early deterioration and premature death. The lungs can easily be kept in good condition, and when we ponder on the beautiful and effective way in which nature has equipped us with a respiratory apparatus and an inexhaustible store of oxygen, surely we must understand the folly of not helping ourselves to what is so vital, yet absolutely free.

Wrong eating and impure air are largely responsible for all kinds of respiratory troubles, from a simple cold to the most aggravated form of pulmonary tuberculosis. Exercise and deep breathing will to a great extent antidote overeating, but there is a limit beyond which the lungs refuse to tolerate this form of abuse.

Experiments have shown that if the carbonic acid gas thrown off daily by an adult male were solidified, it would amount to about seven ounces of solid carbon, which comes from fats, sugars and starches that are burned in the body. It is well to remember that there are various forms of burning or combustion. Rapid combustion is exemplified in stoves and furnaces, where the carbon of coal or wood rapidly and violently unites with oxygen. Slow combustion takes place in the rotting of wood, the rusting of iron and steel and the union of oxygen with organic matter in animal bodies. Both processes are the same, varying only in rapidity and intensity.

People who daily give off seven ounces of carbon are overworking their bodies. They take in too much food and consequently force too great combustion. This forcing has evil effects on the system, for under forced combustion the body is not able to clean itself thoroughly. Some of the soot remains in the flues (the blood-vessels) and is deposited in the various parts of the engine (the body). Result: Hardening, which means loss of elasticity and aging of the body. Aging of the body results in deterioration of the mind. Proper breathing is fine, but unless it is also accompanied by proper eating it does not bring the best results.

The atmospheric air contains about four parts of carbonic acid gas to 10,000 parts of air. The exhaled air becomes quite heavily charged with this gas, about 400 to 500 parts in 10,000. It does not take long before the air in a closed, occupied room is so heavily charged with this gas and so poor in oxygen that its constant rebreathing is detrimental. The blood stream becomes poisoned, which immediately depresses the physical and mental powers. Warning is often given by a feeling of languor and perhaps a slight headache. People accustom themselves to impure air so that they apparently feel no bad effects, but this is always at the expense of health. The senses may be blunted, but the evil results always follow. To keep a house sealed up as tightly as possible in order to keep it warm saves fuel bills, but the resultant bodily deterioration and disease cause enough discomfort and result in doctor bills which more than offset this saving. It is poor economy.

A constant supply of the purest air obtainable must be furnished to the lungs; otherwise the blood becomes so laden with poison that health, in its best and truest sense, is impossible.

The air should be inhaled through the nose. It does not matter much how it is exhaled. The nose is so constructed that it fits the air for the lungs. The inspired air is often too dry, dusty and cold. The normal nose remedies all these defects. The mucous membrane in the nasal passages contains cilia, which catch the dust. The nasal passages are very tortuous so that during its journey through them the air is warmed and takes up moisture.

Habitual mouth breathing is one of the causes of the hardening and toughening of the mucous membrane of the respiratory passages, for the mouth does not arrest the irritating substances floating in the air, nor does it sufficiently warm and moisten the inspired air. Irritation produces inflammation and this in turn causes thickening of the membranes. Then it is very easy to acquire some troublesome affliction such as asthma. Very cold air is irritating, but the passage through the nose warms it sufficiently.

The evil results of mouth breathing are well seen in children, in whom it raises the roof of the mouth and brings the lateral teeth too close together. Then the dentists have to correct the deformity and the children are forced to suffer protracted inconvenience. This mouth breathing is mostly due to wrong feeding, especially overfeeding, which causes swelling of the mucous membrane, thus impeding the intake of the air through the nose and forcing it through the mouth. The chief curative measure is obvious. Cut down the child's food supply and give food of better quality. Remember that children should not be fat.

Normal breathing is rhythmical, with a slight rise of the abdomen and chest during inspiration and a slight falling during expiration. Watch a sleeping baby, and you will understand what is meant. The ratio of breathing to the beating of the heart is about one to four or five. Whatever accelerates the heart causes more rapid breathing and vice versa. Breathing is practically automatic, and were we living under natural conditions we should need to pay no attention to it, but inasmuch as our mode of life prevents the full use of the lungs a little intelligent consideration is necessary to attain full efficiency.

The body should be left as free as possible by the clothes and especially is this true of the chest and waist line. Women sin much against themselves in this respect. Most of them find it absolutely necessary for their mental welfare to constrict the lower part of the chest and the waist line a great part of the time, for really it would not do to be out of fashion. The statue of Venus de Milo is generally considered to represent the highest form of female beauty and perfection in sculptural art. If living women would consent to remain beautiful, instead of being slaves to fashion, it would be much better for themselves and for the race. A corseted woman can not breathe properly, even if she can introduce her hand between the body and her corset to prove that she is not constricted. The natural curves of women are more graceful than those produced by the corset. It would be an easy matter to give the breasts sufficient support, if they need support, without constricting the body, and then take enough exercise to keep the waist and abdomen firm and in shape to accord with a normal sense of what is beautiful and proper.

Woman does right in being as good looking as possible, and it would do man no harm to imitate her in this, for truly, "Beauty is its own excuse for being." But beauty and fashion seldom go hand in hand. Look at the modes which were the fashion, and you will be compelled to say that many of them are offensive to people of good taste. American women should cease imitating the caprice of the women of the underworld of Paris. There are indications that women are liberating themselves somewhat from the chains of fashions, as well as from other ridiculous things, so let us hope that they will soon be brave enough to look as beautiful as nature allows them to be, both in face and figure.

The lungs, like every other part of the body, become weakened when not used. The chest cavity enlarges during inspiration, but this enlargement is prevented if there is constriction of the lower ribs and the waist. The normal breathing is abdominal. Such breathing is health-imparting. It massages the liver gently with each breath and is mildly tonic to the stomach and the bowels. It truly gives internal exercise. It helps to prevent constipation.

Shallow breathing causes degeneration of lung tissue, and indirectly degeneration of every tissue in the body, for it deprives the blood of enough oxygen to maintain health. It also prevents the internal exercise of the abdominal organs, which is a necessary activity of the normal organism. Shallow breathers only use the upper parts of the lungs. It is not to be wondered at that the lower parts easily degenerate. In pneumonia, for instance, the lower part is usually first affected, and in tuberculosis one often can get the physical indications in the lower part of the lungs posteriorly before they can be found any other place. The upper parts have to be used and consequently they get more exercise and more blood and hence become more resistant. It is well known that when the upper part of the lungs become affected the disease is very grave.

Men, as well as women, are guilty of shallow breathing. Many men are very inactive and their breathing becomes sluggish. This can be remedied by taking vigorous exercise and a few breathing exercises. Because abdominal breathing is the correct way, some physical culturists, who mix the so-called New Thought with their system, advocate exercising and concentrating the mind on the abdomen at the same time. This is unnecessary, for the proper exercises and the right attitude will cause abdominal breathing without giving the abdomen special thought.

Man was evidently intended to earn his food through physical exertion and exercise, and so long as he did this the lungs were compelled to expand. A few running exercises or hill or mountain climbs will suffice to prove the truth of this statement. However, now that man can ride on a street car and earn, or at least get, his daily bread by sitting in an office, it is necessary to exercise a little in order to get good results. The farmer who sits crouched up on a plow, mower or binder also fails to use his lungs, but if he gets out and pitches hay or bundles of grain, he is sure to get what oxygen he needs.

Everyone should get into the habit of breathing deeply several times a day. Upon rising in the morning, go to the open window or out of doors and take at least a dozen slow, deep breaths, inhaling slowly, holding the air in the lungs a few moments and exhaling slowly. This should be repeated noon and night. Every time when one is in the fresh air, it is well to take a few full breaths. By and by the proper breathing will become a habit, to the great benefit of one's health.

There are many breathing exercises, but every intelligent being can make his own exercises, so I shall describe but one. Have the hands hanging at the sides, palms facing each other. Inhale slowly and at the same time bring the arms, which are to be held straight, forward and upward, or outward and upward, carrying them as far up and back over the head as possible. The arm motion is also to be slow. About the time the arms are in the last position a full inspiration has been taken. Hold the position of the arms and the breath a few seconds and then slowly exhale and slowly bring the arms back to the first position. Repeat ten or twelve times. If while one is inhaling and raising the arms, one also slowly rises on the toes and slowly resumes a natural foot position while exhaling, the exercise will be even better.

Hollow-chested young people can attain a good lung capacity and good chest contour in a very reasonable time. Persistence in proper breathing and proper exercise will have remarkable results in even two or three months, and at the same time nature will be painting roses on pallid cheeks. It is easy to increase the chest expansion several inches. Those who expand less than three and one-half inches should not be satisfied until they have gone beyond this mark. Elderly people can also increase their chest expansion and breathing capacity, but it takes more time, for with the years the chest cartilages have a tendency to harden and even to ossify. The less breathing the sooner the ossification comes.

Many people are afraid of night air, for which there is no reason. The absence of sunshine at night does no more harm than it does on cloudy days. During the night, of all times, fresh air is needed, for less is used, and what little is breathed should be of as good quality as circumstances permit. Open the windows wide enough to have the air constantly changing in the bedroom. During the winter it will be necessary to put additional clothes on the bed, for no one can obtain the best of slumbers while chilled. Some may find it a better plan to use artificial heat in the foot of the bed. At any rate, during cold weather better covering is required for the legs and for the feet than for any other part of the body. People with good resistance can sleep in a draught without the least harm, but ordinary people should not sleep in a draught. It is easy to use screens so that the wind does not blow upon the face. If the air is kept stirring in the chamber the sleeper gets enough without being in a current.

Some are in the habit of closing their bedroom windows and doors at night and opening them for a thorough airing during the day. If the bedrooms must be closed, close them during the day and open them wide at night, for that is when the pure air is needed. It does not make much difference whether they are open or closed while being unoccupied. It is actually sickening to enter some bedrooms and be compelled to breathe the foul air.

When people are ill the rooms should have fresh air entering at all times. Sick people give off more poisons than do those in good health and they need the oxygen to burn up the deposits in the system.

An early morning stroll while most people are in bed is very instructive. It will be found that some houses are shut up as tightly as possible and that only a few are properly ventilated. A person who insists on keeping his window open in winter is often looked upon as a freak. What is the result of this close housing? The first result is that the blood is unable to obtain the required amount of oxygen and is poisoned by the rebreathing of the air in the room. In the morning the sleeper wakes feeling only half rested, and it takes a cup of coffee or something else to produce complete awakening. The evil results are cumulative, and after a while the bad habit of breathing impure air at night will be a great factor in building disease of some kind.

One reason why some are so afraid of fresh air, especially at night, is that they become so autotoxemic through bad habits, especially improper eating habits, that a slight draught causes them to sneeze and often catch cold and they believe that the fresh air causes the irritation. This is not so. The irritability comes from within, not from without.

After becoming accustomed to good ventilation at night it is almost impossible to enter into restful slumbers in a stuffy room.

Savages are singularly free from respiratory diseases, and the reason is without doubt that they do not house themselves closely. In some parts of the world they fear to let civilized men enter their abodes, for they may bring respiratory diseases.

Not only the homes, but public places, such as street cars, theaters, schools and churches are too often poorly ventilated. Sleeping, or rather dozing in church is so common that it is a matter of jest. My experience has been that drowsiness comes not from the dullness of sermons, but from the impossibility of getting a breath of good air in many churches.

Please remember that exhaled air is excretory matter, and that it is both unclean and unwholesome to consume it over and over again.

Draughts do not cause colds. Cold air does not cause colds. Wet clothes do not cause colds: These things may be minor contributory factors, but the body must be in poor condition before one can catch cold. Colds are generally caught at the table. Lack of fresh air also helps to produce colds, as well as other diseases.

The tendency in our country is to heat buildings too much. Europeans are both surprised and uncomfortable when they first enter our dwellings or public meeting places. The temperature in a dwelling should not be forced above seventy degrees Fahrenheit by means of artificial heating. The temperature required depends very much upon one's mental attitude and habits. Those who take enough exercise have good circulation of the blood in the extremities, and therefore do not need so much artificial heat. The best heating is from within.

CHAPTER XXIV.

SLEEP.

A young baby should sleep almost all the time, and it will if intelligently cared for. Overfeeding is the bane of the baby's life and is the cause of most of its restlessness. The first few months the baby should be awake enough to take its food, and then go to sleep again. As it grows older it sleeps less and less.

There is no fixed time for an adult to sleep. The amount varies with different individuals. The idea is quite prevalent that eight hours nightly are necessary. This may be true for some. Many do very well on seven hours' sleep, and even less. The great inventor, Thomas Edison, is said to have had but very little sleep for many years, and it is reported that when interested in some problem he would miss a night or two. Yet he has lived longer than the average individual and is now in good health. Very few have done as much constructive work as he. Many other prominent people have been light sleepers.

As people grow older they require less sleep than they did in youth. It is not uncommon for septuagenarians to sleep but five hours nightly.

Although we can not say how much sleep any individual may require, each person can find out for himself, and this is much better than to try to live by rules, which are often erroneous.

Those who live as they should otherwise and select a definite hour for retiring and adhere to it, except on special occasions, get all the sleep that is necessary. They awake in the morning refreshed, ready to do a good day's work.

During sound sleep all conscious endeavors cease. The vital organs do only enough work to keep the body alive. The breathing is lighter, the circulation is slower and in sound sleep there is no thinking. This letting up in the great activity of body and mind gives an opportunity for the millions of cells, of which the body is composed, to take from the blood what is needed to restore them to normal. During the day many of these cells become worn and weary. At night they recuperate. Hence undisturbed sleep is very important.

Many believe that "early to bed and early to rise" is the proper way, that the hours of sleep before midnight are more refreshing and invigorating than those after. This is merely a belief, perhaps a good one. Early retiring leads to regularity, which is very desirable. Late retiring often means loose mental and physical habits. Those who are regular about their time of retiring and live well otherwise feel refreshed whether they go to bed early or late. Children should always retire early, otherwise they do not get enough sleep. The night is the natural sleeping time for most creatures, as well as for man. This is a heritage of ages. There was no artificial illumination during the stone age. Man could do nothing during the darkness, so he rested. However, those who must work at night find no trouble in sleeping during the day. The tendency among men is the same as among animals, to sleep more in winter than in summer, not that more sleep is required, but because the winter nights are longer.

Children should go to bed early. They require more sleep than adults because of the greater cell activity. Also, children who stay up late generally become irritable and nervous.

It is not well to eat immediately before retiring. The sleep following a late meal is generally interrupted, and there is not that feeling of brightness and clearness of mind, with which one should awake, next morning.

Lunching before going to bed is a bad habit. Some believe they must have an apple, or perhaps a glass of milk, before retiring, for they think that this will bring sleep. The body should not be burdened with extra food to digest during the sleeping hours. This time should be dedicated to the restoring of the body, and the blood contains ample material.

Dreaming is largely a bad habit. A normal individual rarely dreams, and then generally following some imprudence. Dreams begin in childhood and are then due principally to excessive food intake. As a producer of nightmares overfeeding has no equal. During adult life dreaming is caused by bad physical and mental conduct, plus the habit which was formed in childhood. Fear, anger, worry, stimulants, too much food, impure air and too warm clothes are some of the causes that produce dreams. Like other bad habits, dreaming is difficult to overcome once it is firmly established. The cure consists in righting one's other bad habits and in not thinking about the dreams. A sleep that is disturbed by dreams is not as sound as it should be and consequently not as refreshing as normal sleep. The conscious mind is not completely at rest and, the subconscious mind is running riot. Normal sleep is complete unconsciousness. This is the sleep of the just and must be earned.

Before retiring all the clothes worn during the day should be removed. The night apparel should be light--cotton, linen or silk. The bed should be comfortable, but not too soft. There should be enough covering to keep the sleeper comfortably warm, but not hot. Those who cover themselves with so many quilts or blankets that they perspire during the night are not properly refreshed. It prevents sound sleep and makes the skin too sensitive. It reduces a person's resistance to climatic changes. The feet should be kept warm, even if necessary to put artificial heat in the foot of the bed. During cold weather the feet and the legs should have more covering than the rest of the body. From the waist up the covering should be rather light.

Sound sleep is dependent on relaxation of mind and body. Those who live the day over after going to bed do not go to sleep quickly or easily. This habit should be overcome. Do business at the business place, during business hours, if you would have the mind fresh. There are days so full of cares that the night does not bring mental relaxation, but those who have begun early in life to practice self-control find these days growing fewer as the years roll by. When they learn their true relationship to the rest of humanity, to the universe and to eternity, they are generally willing and able to let the earth rotate and revolve for a few hours without their personal attention. They realize that worry and anxiety waste time and energy.

Many complain that they can not sleep. This they repeat to themselves and to others many times a day. At night they ask themselves why they can not sleep. They do it so often that it becomes a powerful negative suggestion frequently strong enough to prevent their going to sleep. It is an obsession. Real insomnia exists only in the mind of the sufferer. Every physician, sooner or later, has experience with people who say that they can not sleep. The doctors who give such patients sleeping powders or potions make a grave mistake. These drugs are taken at the expense of some of the physical structures, and the day of settlement always comes. Perhaps it will find the patient with bankrupted nerves or a failing heart. To be effective, the size of the dose must be increased from time to time. At last the result will be some disease, either physical or mental.

Those who insist that they "do not sleep at all," or that they sleep "but a few minutes" each night, sleep a few hours, but they make themselves believe that they do not sleep. We are compelled to sleep, and even those who "do not sleep at all" can not remain awake indefinitely.

Those who are troubled with the no-sleep obsession will soon realize that they sleep as well as others if they cease thinking and talking so much about the subject. I have seen people suffering from this bad habit recover in one week. Those who have been taking drugs to induce sleep generally have a few bad nights when they give them up, after which the nervous storm subsides and sleep becomes normal. All drugs should be discarded. The physician who understands more about the working of nature than about the giving of drugs will have the best success in these cases. Soothing sleep always comes to people possessed of a controlled mind in a healthy body.

If the day has been exhausting and the nerves are so alive and wrought up that sleep will not come, do not allow the mind to delve into worry about it. Do not say to yourself: "I wish I could sleep. Why can't I sleep?" Such fretful thinking produces mental tension, which drives sleep away. Instead, say to yourself: "I am very comfortable. I am having a refreshing rest. It does not matter whether I sleep or not." By all means relax the body. Choose a comfortable position and remain quiet, having the muscles relaxed. It is remarkable how soon a relaxed body brings tranquility to a disturbed mind. Let a man in pugnacious mood relax his face and his fists and in a very short time his anger vanishes. It makes no difference whether a person sleeps eight hours on a certain night. If he is fairly regular about going to bed he will get enough sleep. Those who realize this truth do not complain of insomnia.

Most people who think much have an occasional night when an idea takes such strong possession of the brain and demands so forcibly to be put into proper shape, that they can not sleep. Under such circumstances it is as well to to get up and work out the idea. Three or four nights like that in the course of a year will do no harm.

People rarely sleep well when lying on the back. If the theory of evolution is correct, we were not intended to lie on our backs during sleep. A good position is to lie on the right side, the right leg being anterior to the left, both being flexed. Another position that is restful to many is to lie on the abdomen, the arms extended away from the body.

The breathing should be entirely nasal. It will not be nasal if there is obstruction in the nose. A healthy person who breathes through his mouth at night must use autosuggestion to overcome the habit. He should suggest to himself, "I will breathe through the nose; I will keep my lips together." If he persists in this, closes the mouth when he goes to sleep, in time the mouth-breathing will cease, and with it the disagreeable habit of snoring. The harmfulness of mouth-breathing is explained in another chapter.

At all times the bedroom should be well ventilated. Some people are in the habit of sleeping in unventilated bedrooms, but upon rising in the morning they throw the windows open and give the room a good airing. The ventilation does not do much good except when there is someone in the room. During the day the bedroom could be closed with very little harm ensuing, though it is best to have it sunned and aired as much as possible.

The sleeping porch is excellent. Outdoor sleeping is all right and it is not a modern fad. Where Benjamin Franklin got his information I do not know, but he has this to say about outdoor sleeping: "It is recorded that Methusaleh, who, being the longest liver, may be supposed to have best preserved his health, that he slept always in the open air; for when he had lived five hundred years an angel said to him: 'Arise, Methusaleh, and build thee an house, for thou shalt live five hundred years longer.' But Methusaleh answered, and said: 'If I am to live but five hundred years longer, it is not worth while to build me an house; I will sleep in the air as I have been used to do.'" This may partly account for some of his many years. His alleged conversation with the angel indicates that he was a man of equanimity.

Under ordinary circumstances those who sleep indoors should have one sash of window fully open for each person in the chamber, or more. It is well to have plenty of fresh air, but it is not best to sleep in a draught. When the wind is blowing through the windows it is not necessary to have them wide open, for an aperture of four inches will then give as much fresh air as a sash opening in calmer weather.

It is best to get up promptly upon awakening in the morning. Remaining in bed half asleep is productive of slothfulness. Too much sleeping and dozing make one dull.

Those who overeat require more sleep than moderate people. The sluggishness and sleepiness following a too heavy meal are familiar to all. Animals that do not get food regularly, but are dependent on the vicissitudes of preying for their nourishment, often gorge themselves so that they can not stay awake, but fall into a stupor, which may last for days. Man, who is generally assured of three meals a day, has no excuse for this form of self-abuse, but unfortunately he practices it too often. It is a gross habit, one in which people of refinement will not continue to indulge.

Young children should take a nap each day. They are so active that they need this rest. Adults can with profit take a short nap, not to exceed thirty minutes, after lunch. Those who are nervous owe it to themselves to take a nap. Those who use the brain a great deal will find the midday nap a great restorer. If sleep will not come, they should at least close their eyes and remain relaxed for a short time. A long nap makes one feel stupid.

Those unfortunate people who are addicted to various enslaving drugs, such as cocaine and morphine, often are very light sleepers. They are deteriorating physically, mentally and morally. Such people are ill and are no guides to the needs of healthy people.

Coffee drinking is a destroyer of sound sleep. At first the coffee seems to soothe the nerves, but in a few hours it has the opposite effect. The habitual use of coffee helps to bring on premature nervous instability and physical degeneration.

Sleep is self-regulating. If we are normal otherwise we need give the subject no thought except to select a regular time to go to bed and get up promptly in the morning upon awaking.

It is easy to drive away sleep. Those who wish to enjoy this sweet restorer at its best must be regular.

CHAPTER XXV.

FASTING.

Fasting is one of the oldest of remedial measures known to man, not only for the ills of the body, but for those of the soul. Oriental lore and literature make frequent reference to fasts. From the Bible we learn that Moses, Elijah and Christ each fasted forty days, and no bad effects are recorded.

Addison knew the value of fasting and temperance. He wrote that, "Abstinence well-timed often kills a sickness in embryo and destroys the seeds of a disease." Unfortunately, he did not live as well as he knew how. Hence his brilliant mind had but a short time in which to work and the world is the loser.

Our own great philosopher, Benjamin Franklin, had the same knowledge, for he wrote, "Against disease known, the strongest fence is the defensive virtue, abstinence."

There is much prejudice against fasting, because people do not understand what fasting is and what it accomplishes. Fasting is not starving. To fast is to go without food when the body is in such condition that food can not be properly digested and assimilated. To starve is to go without food when the body is in condition to digest and assimilate food and needs nourishment.

It is quite generally believed that if food is withheld for six or seven days the result will be fatal. Under proper conditions one can go without food for two or three months. Perhaps most people could not do without food for the latter period, but fasts of that duration are on record. Fat people can live on their tissues for a long time before they are reduced to normal weight, and slender ones can live on water for an extended period.

Prolonged fasts should not be taken unless necessary, and then they should be taken under the guidance of someone who has had experience and is possessed of common sense. If a person is fearful or surrounded by others who instill fear into him, he should not take a prolonged fast. The gravest danger during the fast is fear. It takes many weeks to die from lack of food, but fear is capable of killing in a few days, or even in a few hours. The healer who undertakes to direct fasts against the wishes of the patient's friends and relatives, who have more influence than he has, injures himself professionally and throws doubt upon the valuable therapeutic measure he advocates.

The indications that a fast is needed are pain and fever and acute attacks of all kinds of diseases. Some of the more common diseases that call for a complete cessation of eating are: The acute stage of pneumonia, appendicitis, typhoid fever, neuralgia, sciatica, peritonitis, cold, tonsilitis, whooping cough, croup, scarlet fever, smallpox and all other eruptive diseases; colics of kidneys, liver or bowels; all acute alimentary tract disturbances, whether of the stomach or of the bowels.

Sometimes it is necessary to fast in chronic diseases, especially when there is pain, but as a rule chronic diseases yield to proper hygienic and dietetic treatment without a fast, provided they are curable. Here is where many people who advocate fasting go to extremes. A fast is the quickest way out of the trouble, but it is at times very unpleasant. By taking longer time the result can be obtained by proper living and the patient is being educated while he is recovering. In chronic cases it is especially important to eat properly.

The only disease of which I know that seems to be unfavorably influenced by fasting is pulmonary tuberculosis in well advanced stages. Such patients quickly lose weight and strength on a fast, and they have great difficulty in regaining either. Perhaps others have had different experiences and have made observations that do not agree with this, for cases of tuberculosis have been reported cured through fasting. It is well to bear in mind that every case that is diagnosed pulmonary tuberculosis is not tuberculosis. Many supposed-to-be cases of tuberculosis, some of them so diagnosed by most reputable specialists, are nothing more than lung irritation due to the absorption of gas and acid from the digestive tract. When the indigestion is cured, the so-called tuberculosis disappears. These are the only tubercular cases that I have seen benefited by fasts, and the improvement is both quick and sure.

Doubtless tuberculosis in the first stages could be cured by fasting, followed by proper hygienic and dietetic care, for at first tuberculosis is a localized symptom of disordered nutrition. In this stage the disease is no more dangerous than many other maladies that are not considered fatal. The subjects brought to the dissecting table show plainly that a large proportion of them have at some time had pulmonary tuberculosis, the lesions of which were healed, and they afterwards died of some other affliction. However, if a patient is received after the manifestation of profuse night sweats, great flushing of the cheeks, high fever daily, emaciation, expulsion of much mucus from the lungs, and the presence of great lassitude and weakness, the rule is that the nutrition is so badly impaired that nothing will bring the patient back to normal. Under such circumstances fasting hastens death. The family and friends are not reticent about placing the blame on the healer. Moderate feeding will prolong life and add to the comfort of the sufferer. The customary overfeeding hastens the end.

Cancer is said to be cured by fasting, but this is very, very doubtful. It is often difficult to differentiate between cancer and benignant tumors at first. Benignant tumors frequently disappear on a limited diet. I have seen many tumors disappear under rational treatment, without resorting to the knife, but I have never seen an undoubted case of cancer do so, though some of the tumors in question had been diagnosed cancer. Cancers, in the advanced stages, end in the death of the patient in spite of any kind of treatment. By being very careful about the diet, cancer patients can escape nearly all the pain and discomfort that generally accompany this disease. Moderation would prevent nearly every case of cancer, and especially moderation in meat eating. It is a disease that should be prevented, for its cure is very doubtful.

Colds leave in a few days, with no bad after effects, if no food is taken.

Typhoid fever treated rationally from the start generally disappears in from one week to twelve days if nothing but water is given, and fails to develop the severity that it attains under the giving of foods and drugs. There are no complications.

Appendicitis is of longer duration, if it is a severe attack, lasting from two to four weeks, but after the first few days the patient is comfortable, under a no-food, let-alone treatment. Operation is not necessary.

In cases of gall-stones, accompanied by jaundice and colic, it is not necessary to operate. Fasting and bathing will bring the body back to normal in a short time. In such cases it is necessary to give the baths as hot as they can be borne, and prolong them until the body is relaxed.

It would be easy to enumerate many diseases, telling the benefits to be derived from fasting, but these point the way and are sufficient.

The one unfailing symptom of a fast is the loss of weight. This loss is natural and there is nothing alarming about it. As soon as eating is resumed the loss of weight stops. For a while the weight may then remain stationary, but the gain is generally prompt. In time the weight will become normal again.

According to Chosat, the loss sustained by the various tissues in starvation is as follows:

Fat.................... 93 per cent. Blood................... 75 " Spleen.................. 71 "
Pancreas............... 64 " Liver.................. 52 " Muscles................ 43 "
Nervous tissues.......... 2 "

This table was made from animal experimentation, but agrees very well with other observations, except in the loss of blood, which others have found to be less than 20 per cent. It will be noticed that the highest tissue, nervous tissue, is hardly affected, but the lowest tissue, fat, almost disappears.

When an individual needs to fast, his body is suffering from the ingestion of too much food and poor elimination. He overworks his nutrition and overdraws on his nervous energies so much in other lines that the body is unable to throw off the debris which should leave by way of the kidneys, the bowels, the skin and the lungs. He is poisoned by his retained excretions, suffering from what is called autointoxication or self-poisoning. He is filthy internally and needs a cleaning. If he has abused himself so that he lacks the power to assimilate food and throw off waste at the same time, obviously it is proper to stop eating until the lost power is regained. In cases of fever it is a physical crime to eat, for the glands cease secreting the normal juices. The mouth becomes parched for lack of saliva, and the gastric and intestinal juices are not secreted in proper amount or quality. Food eaten under such circumstances is not digested. The internal temperature in fever is above 100 degrees Fahrenheit, and it does not take long for food to decay in such temperature, especially such aliments as milk and broth, which are the favorite foods for fever patients. These alimentary substances are excellent for growing nearly all the germs that are found in the body in disease.

When in pain, it is harmful to eat, for the secretions are then perverted and digestion is interfered with. All violent emotions, such as hatred, jealousy, and anger, mean that no food should be taken until the body has had the opportunity to relax and regain some of its tone. Such emotions do not thrive so well in healthy individuals as among the sick, but then perfect health is a rarity.

When going without food people are subject to various symptoms, which depend as much on the temperament as on the physical conditions. A hysterical woman can scare inexperienced attendants into doing her will by her antics. She may make them believe that she is dying. On the other hand, well balanced, fearless people can fast for weeks with very little annoyance. Fasting is not always pleasant and there are a number of symptoms that are often present.

The faster loses weight, at first often as much as two pounds a day. This is mostly water. After the first ten days the loss may be but one-half of a pound, or less, per day. The loss of weight is greatest in heavy people and in those who have high fevers.

The tongue becomes badly coated, and the breath foul, showing that the mucous membrane is busy throwing out waste. The tongue remains coated until the system is clean, and then it clears off. Most people feel weak when they attempt to walk or work, but they feel strong when resting. Others, who are badly food-poisoned, gain strength as the system eliminates the harmful substances from the body. For a day or two the craving for food may be quite insistent and persistent. Then hunger generally leaves and does not return until the tongue is clean. The mind becomes clearer as the body becomes cleaner. This benefit to the spirit, or the soul, has been recognized by religious organizations for centuries.

A little discharge of blood from the bowels at first should cause no alarm. In some cases a great deal of yellow mucus is thrown into the lower bowel. The liver at times throws off so much bile that it makes the patient alarmed. This should cause no uneasiness. When the bile is forced upward into the stomach it is very disagreeable. The discharges from the bowels are often very dark.

There is a tendency toward chilliness, especially to have cold hands and feet. Skin eruptions and heart palpitations are occasional symptoms. Nervous, irritable and fearful people have symptoms too numerous to mention. The more they are sympathized with the worse they become.

Many medical men have misinterpreted the symptoms of the fast, and hence they have condemned the procedure. They see the foul coating on the tongue, the loss of weight and at times peculiar mental manifestations. They can smell the foul breath and the disagreeable odor from the skin and from the bowel discharges. These they interpret as signs of physical deterioration and degeneration. These manifestations indicate that the entire body is cleansing itself, throwing out impurities that have accumulated, because the system has had so much work to do that it has lacked the power to be self-cleansing. Nothing is needed to prove this fact except to continue the fast until the odors disappear and the tongue becomes clean.

The bad odors given off by the body resemble the odors in severe fevers with much wasting, and hence they alarm those who have had little or no experience with protracted fasts. These odors are often bad at the end of about one week of fasting, though there is no fixed period for their appearance. They should cause no alarm for they simply indicate that the body is cleansing itself, and that is exactly what is desired. Under proper conditions I have neither seen nor heard of a fatality coming from a short fast. Those who are in such physical shape that they will die if fasted from five to ten days would die if they were fed.

Another symptom that may alarm the attendant is the lowered blood pressure. This is natural and should cause no anxiety. Eating and drinking keep the blood pressure up. When the food intake is decreased, the blood pressure is reduced. When the food intake is stopped, the blood pressure is still further reduced. This fact should give the intelligent healer the hint to reduce the food intake in such abnormal conditions as arteriosclerosis and apoplexy. During prolonged fasts the blood pressure generally becomes quite low.

Some fasting people can continue with light work, and when they are able to do this, it is best, for it keeps them from thinking about themselves all the time. If there is a lack of energy, dispense with work and vigorous exercise. In acute diseases there is no choice. One is compelled to cease laboring. In chronic diseases it depends on the patient and the adviser.

Dismiss fear from the mind and do not discuss the fast or any of the symptoms with anyone except the adviser. It is best not to tell any outsiders about the fast, for the public has some queer ideas on the subject. If you are afraid, or if you have to fight with neighbors, friends, relatives, or perhaps with the health authorities, as sometimes happens, it is better not to take the fast.

Drink all the water desired. At first the more one drinks the more quickly the system cleanses itself. A glass of water every hour during the day, or even every half hour is all right. The water may be warm or cold, but it should not be ice-cold nor should it be hot. Both extremes produce irritation.

In acute inflammation of the stomach, nothing should be given by mouth. Small quantities of water may be given by rectum every two or three hours. In appendicitis only very small quantities of water are to be given by mouth at first, until the acute symptoms have subsided. Large quantities of fluid may excite violent peristalsis with resulting pain. In all eases of nausea, give nothing by mouth, not even water, until the nausea is gone. Symptoms are nature's sign language, and when properly interpreted they tell us what to do and what not to do.

Even though there be no thirst or desire for water, some should be taken. If it can be taken by mouth give at least a glassful every two hours, not necessarily all at once. Some are so sensitive that one-half of a glass of water is all they can tolerate. If the stomach objects to water, give it by rectum.

Always do this in cases of much nausea. After a few days the water intake may be reduced.

Take a quick sponge bath every day and if there is any inclination toward chilliness, the water should be tepid or warm. Follow with a few minutes of dry towel friction. People who are overweight, with good heart and kidney action, can take prolonged hot baths, if they wish. An olive oil rub immediately after the bath, about twice a week, is grateful. However, this is not necessary.

The colon is to be washed out every day. No definite amount of water can be prescribed. Occasionally enemas are taken under difficulties, for some cramp when water is introduced into the bowel. Those who are not accustomed to enemas should use water about 100 degrees Fahrenheit. One quart is a small enema. Two quarts make a fairly large one. Introduce the water, lie still for a few minutes and then allow it to pass out. If the bowels are very foul, use two or three washings. If there is much fermentation, use some soda in the water. Salt, about a tablespoonful to two quarts of water, stimulates the bowels, but its disadvantage is that it draws water from the intestinal walls, thus robbing the blood of a part of its fluid. The same is true of glycerin. Perhaps the least harmful ingredient that can be put into the water to stimulate action is enough pure castile soap to render the water opaque. The soap, however, has a tendency to wash away too much of the mucus which lubricates the bowel. On the whole, nothing is better than plain water. If it gives good results use nothing else.

Those who are very sensitive and weak often find that the expulsion of water from the bowel not only further weakens them, but causes pain. In such cases Dr. Hazzard recommends a rectal tube (not a colon tube), which is very good, for it allows the emptying of the bowel without any cramping. The tube is to be inserted about six inches.

To take the enema, assume either the knee-chest position (kneeling with the shoulders close to the floor) or lie on the right side with the hips elevated. These positions allow water to flow into colon by aid of gravity.

When it is necessary to supply liquid to the body by rectum, simply introduce a pint or less of plain water, moderately warm. Repeat as often as necessary to keep away thirst, which will rarely be more than every three hours.

Keep the body warm at all times. If it is difficult to keep warm, go to bed and use enough covers, having the windows open enough to supply fresh air. At night use artificial heat in the foot of the bed. If hot-water bottles, warm bricks or stones are used, they should be quite large; otherwise they become cold by two or three o'clock in the morning, when heat is most needed. If a large receptacle, such as a jug, is used to keep the water in, the bed clothes are lifted off the patient's feet, and this is often a great relief.

No special food is suited to break all fasts on. It is necessary to begin with plain food in moderation. Overeating or eating of indigestible food at this time may result in sickness and even in death. If the faster lacks self-control, the food should be brought to him in proper quantities by the attendant.

If the fast has lasted but two or three days, no special precautions are necessary, except that the first few meals should be smaller than usual.

As indiscretions in eating compel nearly all fasts it is necessary to do a little better than previously, or the fast must be repeated. It is best to live so that fasts are not necessary.

If the fast has been prolonged it is best to begin feeding liquid foods. What shall we feed? That depends on the patient and circumstances. The juice of the concord grape is not good for it ferments too easily. Many of those who are compelled to fast or else die have been so food-poisoned, and their digestive organs have been in such horrible condition for years that they have been unable to eat acid fruits. This is especially true of those who consume large quantities of starch. Sometimes they are unable to eat fruit for a while after the fast. At other times the irritability of the digestive organs disappears while food is withheld. For such people broths and milk may be employed.

The juice of oranges, pineapples, California grapes, cherries, blackberries or tomatoes may be given. The tomatoes may be made into broth and strained, but nothing is to be added to this broth except salt. Stout people should do well on fruit juices. They are not to be so highly recommended for very thin, nervous people, for fruit juices are both thinning and cooling. Milk is very useful, and may be given either sweet or clabbered or in the form of buttermilk.

Thin, nervous people can safely be given broths, preferably of lamb, mutton or chicken. Trim away all the fat, grind up the lean meat, and allow it to simmer (not boil) until all the juices are extracted from the meat. Strain and put away to cool. When cold, skim off the fat. Then warm the broth and serve. This broth is not to be seasoned while it is being cooked, but a little salt may be added when it is ready to serve. To one pound of lean meat there should be about one quart of broth. A teacupful to begin with is enough for a meal, and it is often necessary to give less than this. The gravest mistake is to be in a hurry about returning to full meals. The remarks about moderate feeding also apply to milk and fruit juices.

Ordinarily, fasts are not broken on starchy foods, but this may be done at times to advantage, especially in cases that have been accustomed to large quantities of starch and but little of the fresh raw foods. The starch must, however, be in an easily digestible state and should be in the form of a very thin gruel made of oatmeal or whole wheatmeal. It should be cooked four to six hours and dressed with nothing but a little salt. A few can break the fast on a full meal without any bad results, but most people can not do it without suffering and the results may be fatal. So it is a safe rule to break the fast on simple liquid food, taken in moderation.

Four or five days after breaking the fast, one should be able to eat the ordinary foods. The following is a suggestion of the manner in which to feed immediately after a fast of about two weeks:

First day: Tomato broth once; mutton broth twice.

Second day: Breakfast, orange juice. Lunch, buttermilk. Dinner, sliced tomatoes.

Third day: Breakfast, buttermilk. Lunch, salad of lettuce and tomatoes, dressed with salt. Dinner, poached egg, celery.

Fourth day: Breakfast, baked apple and milk. Lunch, toasted bread and butter. Dinner, lamb chops, stewed green peas, celery.

If a meal causes distress, omit the next one and continue omitting meals until comfort and ease have returned. If the digestion is very weak, or if the illness has been protracted, do not feed solids as soon as recommended above. In all cases it is necessary to exercise self-control, moderation and common sense.

The meals must be moderate. Gradually increase until the amount of food taken is sufficient to do the necessary bodily rebuilding. The longer the fast, the more care should be exercised in the beginning. It is no time to experiment.

If the fast is to be of permanent benefit it is necessary to learn how to eat properly afterwards, and to put this knowledge into practice. This is the most important part to emphasize, yet all the books I have read on the subject have failed to pay any attention to it. In nearly every case the fast is necessary because of repeated mistakes in eating and drinking. Those mistakes built bodily ills in the first place and if the faster goes back to them they will do it again. The disease does not always take on the same type as it did in the first place, but it is the same old disease. During a fast there is recuperation because the body has a chance to become clean, and a clean body can not long remain unbalanced, provided there are no organic faults. By making mistakes in eating after the fast is over, the body again becomes foul and full of debris and that means more disease. Perhaps it may not require more than one-third as much abuse to cause a second break-down as it did to bring about the first one.

Some people fast repeatedly, and are somewhat proud of it. They should be ashamed of the fact that they must fast time after time, for it shows either ignorance or a weak, undeveloped will power. The fast should teach every intelligent being that it is an emergency measure, and emergencies are but seldom encountered in a well regulated life.

Food debauches following fasts should be avoided. A little will power properly applied will prevent them. Gross eating may compel another fast. We must eat and it is better to eat so that we can take sustenance regularly than to be compelled to go without food at various intervals. He who is moderate in his eating, uses a fair degree of intelligence in the selection of his food, is temperate in other ways and considerate and kind in his dealings with others will not be ill.

A fast is efficacious in clearing up a brain that is unable to work well because it is bathed in unclean blood. It is remarkable how well the brain works when the stomach is not overworked. Overfeeding the body causes underfeeding of the brain. On a correct diet the brain is efficient and clear and able to bear sustained burdens.

There is no question but that a fast, followed by a light diet, containing less of the heavily starchy and proteid foods and more of the succulent vegetables and fresh fruits, with their cleansing juices and health-imparting salts, would result in the recovery of over one-half of the insane. Most of them are suffering functionally and here the outlook is very hopeful. Christ cured a lunatic "by prayer and fasting." Proper feeding would work wonders in prisons. It would also be very beneficial for wayward girls and young men who are passion's slaves. St. Peter recommended fasting as an aid to morality, which is another evidence of the profundity of his wisdom.

How long should a fast last? Until its object has been accomplished. It is rarely necessary to fast a month, but sometimes it is advisable to continue the fast for forty days, or even longer. If the fast is taken on account of pain, continue until the pain is gone. If for fever, until there is no more fever. In chronic cases it is not always necessary to continue the fast until the tongue is clean. When the patient is free from pain and fever and comfortable in every way, start feeding lightly. People who are thin and have sluggish nutrition, one symptom of which is dirty-gray mucous membrane in mouth and throat, should not be fasted any longer than it is absolutely necessary, for they generally react slowly and poorly.

If people would miss a meal or two or three as soon as they begin to feel bad, no long fasts would be necessary, because when the system first begins to be deranged it very quickly rights itself when food is withheld. It is impossible for a serious disease to develop in a fasting person, unless he is in an exceptionally bad physical condition at the beginning of the fast, for when food is withheld there is nothing for disease to feed upon. No new disease can originate during a fast.

Fasts often bring people back to health, who can not recover through any other means known to man, unless it be eating almost nothing--a semi-fast. Occasionally a patient dies while on a long fast or immediately thereafter, but please remember that millions die prematurely on this earth every year who never missed their meals for one day. Also remember that those who go on prolonged fasts are generally "hopeless cases," who have been given up to die by medical men. People who fast generally become comfortable, so why envy a few men and women an easy departure when they are no longer able to live, and why heap undeserved censure on those who are doing their best to ease the sufferers by means of our most valuable therapeutic measure, fasting?

There is much prejudice against fasting, but a calm study of the facts will remove this. Typhoid fever, conventionally treated, often proves fatal in 15 per cent. or more of the cases and those who survive have to undergo a long, uncomfortable illness which often leaves them so weakened and with such degenerated bodies that the end is frequently a matter of a few months or years. Pneumonia and tuberculosis find a favorable place to develop and in these cases prove very fatal. On the other hand, cases of typhoid treated by the fast, and the other hygienic measures necessary, recover in a short time, there are no evil sequels and the body is in better condition than it was before the onset of the disease. I have never seen a fatality in a properly treated case, and the mortality is conspicuous by its absence. It is the same in curable chronic diseases. Where feeding and medicating add to the ills, fasting with proper living afterwards brings health.

It is also well to remember that where one individual dies while fasting (not from the effects of fasting, but from the disease for which the fast was begun), perhaps one hundred thousand starve because they have too much to eat. Silly as this may sound, it is the truth, and this is s the explanation: Overfeeding causes digestive troubles and a breakdown of the assimilative and excretory processes. The more food that is taken while this condition exists the less nourishment is extracted from it. The food ferments pathologically, instead of physiologically, and poisons the body. The more that is eaten under the circumstances, the worse is the poisoning and at last the tired body wearily gives up the fight for existence, perhaps after a long chronic ailment has been suffered, or perhaps during the attack of an acute disease. The chief cause of death is too much food.

Avicena, the great Arabian physician, treated by means of prolonged fasts.

For the benefit of those who fear the effects of fasts of a few days' duration a few quotations are given from various sources:

"My next marked case is a wonderful illustration of the self-feeding power of the brain to meet an emergency, and a revelation, also, of the possible limitations of the starvation period. This was the case of a frail, spare boy of four years, whose stomach was so disorganized by a drink of solution of caustic potash that not even a swallow of water could be retained. He died on the seventy-fifth day of his fast, with the mind clear to the last hour, and with apparently nothing of the body left but bones, ligaments, and a thin skin; and yet the brain had lost neither weight nor functional clearness.

"In another city a similar accident happened to a child of about the same age, in whom it took three months for the brain to exhaust entirely the available body-food."--Dr. E. H. Dewey.

This shows the groundlessness of the fear parents have of allowing their children to fast when necessary. It is beneficial for even the babies who need it. In the cases quoted above the conditions were very unfavorable, for the children were suffering from the effects of lye burns, yet they lived without food seventy-five and ninety days, respectively. If necessary, deprive the children of food, and keep them warm. Then comfort yourself with the fact that they are being treated humanely and efficiently.

Dr. Linda Burfield Hazzard, in the latest edition of her book, Fasting for the Cure of Disease, states that she has treated almost two thousand five hundred people by this method, the fasts varying in duration from eight to seventy five days, many of them being over a month. Sixteen of her patients have died while fasting and two on a light diet. This is far from being a mortality of 1 per cent. When the fact is taken into consideration that the people she treated were of the class for whom the average medical man can do nothing the mortality is surprisingly small. However, she has lost a few, and as she is a fighter for her beliefs the prejudice against her and her method of treating disease have proved strong enough to cause her to be imprisoned. Dr. Hazzard has perhaps the widest experience with fasting of any mortal, living or dead. Her book is well worth reading.

Upton Sinclair has also written a book on this subject, entitled the Fasting Cure. He writes from the viewpoint of an intelligent layman whose observations are not very extensive. The book contains many good ideas. This is from page fifty-seven:

"The longest fast of which I had heard when my article was written was seventy eight days; but that record has since been broken, by a man named Richard Fausel. Mr. Fausel, who keeps a hotel somewhere in North Dakota, had presumably partaken too generously of the good cheer intended for his guests, for he found himself at the inconvenient weight of three hundred and eighty-five pounds. He went to a sanatorium in Battle Creek and there fasted for forty days (if my recollection serves me), and by dint of vigorous exercise meanwhile, he got rid of one hundred and thirty pounds. I think I never saw a funnier sight than Mr. Fausel at the conclusion of this fast, wearing the same pair of trousers that he had worn at the beginning of it. But the temptations of hotel-keepers are severe, and when he went back home, he found himself going up in weight again. This time he concluded to do the job thoroughly, and went to Macfadden's place in Chicago, and set out upon a fast of ninety days. That is a new record--though I sometimes wonder if it is quite fair to call it 'fasting' when a man is simply living upon an internal larder of fat."

Bernarr Macfadden has also written considerable about fasting. C. C. Haskell is an advocate and director of such treatment. Many physicians employ this healing method. Some day the entire medical profession will realize the worth of fasting as a curative agent.

As a reminder, please allow me to repeat: When reading and studying about the subject of fasting, do not think of it as a complete cure, for those who return to their improper mode of living will again build disease. After the fast, live right.

The efficient body is clean internally. An unclean skin is bad. A foul alimentary tract is worse. But the worst of all is a foul condition of all the tissues, including the blood-stream, a condition in which much of the body's waste is stored up, instead of being excreted.

If such a condition can not be remedied through moderation and simplicity in eating, the only thing that will prove of value is temporary abstinence.

It would be an easy matter to enumerate many long fasts, such as that of Dr. Tanner, who proved to an astonished country that fasting for a month or more is not fatal, but on the contrary may be beneficial. Or we could cite cases like the fasts carried on by classes under the direction of Bernarr Macfadden. Or we could refer to the experiments of Professors Fisher and Chittenden of Yale.

However, we will only look into one more case, that of Dr. I. J. Eales, whose fast created considerable interest several years ago. The doctor was too heavy, so he decided to take a fast to reduce his weight, also for scientific purposes. For thirty days he lived on nothing but water with an occasional glass of lemonade and one cup of coffee. At the end of thirty days he broke his fast on a glass of malted milk.

The doctor worked hard during all this period, losing weight all the time, being thirty pounds lighter at the end of his fast than at the beginning. However, he did not lose strength, being able to do as much work and lift as heavy weights at the end of the fast as at the beginning. Anyone who is much over weight can with benefit do as the doctor did, for the body will use the stored up fat to produce heat and energy. This fast is fully detailed in Dr. Eales' book called Healthology.

Fasting is the quickest way to produce internal cleanliness, which is health. When the system is clean the cravings, longings and appetites are not so strong as when the body is full of poisons. For this reason a fast is the best way to destroy the cravings for tobacco, coffee, tea, alcohol and other habit-forming drugs. If, after the fast is over, the individual lives moderately and simply, and is fully determined not to return to the use of these drugs, a permanent cure will be the reward. However, it is very easy to drift back into the old habits. A permanent cure requires that there be no compromise, no saying, "I shall do it this time, but never again." Once the old habit is resumed, it is almost certain to be continued.

CHAPTER XXVI.

ATTITUDE OF PARENT TOWARD CHILD.

Healthy, happy children are the greatest of all rewards. All parents can have such children, and it is a duty they owe themselves, the children and the race. It is a most pleasant duty, for the returns are far greater than the cost.

In order to have first-class children parents must be in good physical condition and be controlled mentally. Chaotic parents can not have orderly children. The young people learn quickly from their elders and they usually take after one of the parents. They intuitively learn what they can do and what they can not do and how to get their way while we consider them too young to have any understanding.

Therefore it is important that their first impressions are correct. Begin to train the child in the way it should go from the day of birth. The first training will have to do with feeding and sleeping. These points are covered more fully in the next chapter. They are touched upon here to give them emphasis.

Feed the child three times a day, but never wake it to be fed. If you give the three feeds, the child will soon become accustomed to them and wake when it is time. If the child squirms and frets, it may be uncomfortable from being overfed or it may be thirsty. Offer it water but not food.

Let the child alone. Do not bounce it or carry it about. During the first few months the baby needs heat, nourishment and rest, and should have no excitement. It should not be treated as a plaything. After a few months it begins to take notice of things and then you can have much fun with it.

The right kind of love consists in doing what is necessary for the infant and no more.

Obedience to the reasonable requests of the parents is of the greatest importance in the successful raising of children. Parents should realize this even before the children are born. From the first, be firm, though gentle, with the little ones. Children should be so trained that when they are requested to do a thing, they do it immediately without any repetition. This will save both them and the parents many an unhappy hour.

The lives of many parents and many children are made miserable from lack of a little parental firmness at the start.

There are many little graces that are not vital, yet they are important, and these should be taught children early, for then they become second nature. Among these are good table manners. Ungainly table manners have no bearing on the health, but they give an unfavorable impression to others. We are partly judged by the presence or absence of such little graces.

Training children is like training trees. A sapling can be made to grow in the desired way, but after a few years it will not respond to training. The period of infancy is plastic, and then is the time to plant the seeds in the child's mind and teach good habits.

It is not difficult to train the children. If the parents are orderly and firm, instead of wavering, the children almost intuitively fall into line. Teach them to obey and they will later be able to command intelligently and considerately.

The babies are helpless at first. This softens the hearts of the parents toward them until they become very indulgent. Indulging and pampering children are bad for them. Kindness consists in doing for them what is for their good, which is not always what they desire.

If the children are properly trained at first, they need very little training later on.

CHAPTER XXVII.

CHILDREN.

Statistics are generally very dry and uninteresting, but at times they take on a tragic interest, and the importance of the few submitted here is so great that they should command careful attention.

The definite figures used are taken from the Mortality Statistics, United States Census, and they cover the year 1912, which is the last year for which we have definite information. Reliable mortality statistics are given only in a part of the country, which is not to our credit. The population is reported in the volume as 92,309,348. The registration area, which is the area giving mortality statistics, contains 53,843,896 people. In this area the total deaths are as follows:

Under one year.............. 154,373 Under ten years............. 235,262

Taking it for granted that the infant and child mortality among the unregistered people is the same, we get the following number of deaths annually among children in the United States, in round numbers:

Under one year.............. 280,000 Under ten years............. 425,000

This is a very conservative estimate and 300,000 is usually given as the number of deaths annually among babies under the age of one year.

Even under ideal conditions a baby would occasionally die, but the deaths would be so rare that they would be the cause of surprised comment. Some become parents who have no right to be, and they bring children into the world who are not physically fit to survive, and these generally die within a few days or weeks of birth. However, these babies are but a small minority and at least ninety-nine out of a hundred should survive. Not one baby born physically fit would die if intelligently cared for, and the fact that each year we lose over one-fourth million infants under one year of age in the United States is an indictment of our lives and intelligence, and a challenge to better our ways.

Every child that is brought into the world should be given an opportunity to live. This is far from the case today. Children are so handicapped that they are stunted in body and blunted in mind, if they survive.

Suppose that every ten years an army of 4,250,000 men and women between the ages of twenty and thirty were destroyed at one time in this country! The indignation, sorrow and horror would be so great that a means would soon be found to end the periodic slaughter.

But we allow this many children under ten to be destroyed every ten years. The slaughter of the innocents does not bring forth much protest, because we are so used to it, and the babies go one by one, all over the country. The procession to the grave gives rise to this thought: "The little one is better off. Now he will suffer no more. It is the will of Providence." This is a libel on Providence, for this enormous mortality is due to parental mistakes, mistakes made mostly through ignorance, but blamable all the same. It behooves parents to obtain knowledge that will prevent such costly and fatal errors. Nature's law is the same as man's rule in this that ignorance of the law excuses no one. The results are the same whether we err knowingly or ignorantly.

It is difficult to teach people to treat their babies properly, because nearly all the information on the subject is so erroneous. When a teacher brings forth the truth but few accept it, for the vast majority are on the other side. Those parents who accept the truth find it difficult, to put it into practice, for every hand is against them. It takes more strength of character and moral courage than the average individual possesses to withstand the criticism of neighbors, friends, relatives and medical advisers.

The few who have the courage of their convictions and the right knowledge reap a rich harvest. They have babies who are well. They see their children grow up with sound bodies and clear minds. They are saved much of the worry which is the lot of parents of children raised according to conventional standards. Last, but by no means least, they have the satisfaction of giving to the race individuals who are better than their parents or the grandparents. There is much opportunity for human improvement, and the improvement will take place automatically, if we do not prevent it by going contrary to nature.

Healthy babies spring from normal, healthy parents. If they can have normal grandparents, so much the better, but inasmuch as we can not alter the past, let us give our attention to the present. If we take care of the present, the future will bring forth a population of healthy parents and grandparents, and then the babies will have full opportunity. The past has great influence, for the child of today is heir of the past, modified by the present. He who influences the present leaves his mark on the future. As individuals we do not usually accomplish much during a lifetime, but if we influence our time for the better it is hard to tell where the improvement will cease or what will be the aggregate result. A truth imparted to others acts much like a pebble cast into the water. Its influence is felt in ever widening circles.

Infancy and youth are plastic. Both body and mind are susceptible to surrounding influences. If the heredity is unfavorable it can be largely modified by favorable environments. If a child is born of unhealthy parents, but without any serious defect, and is intelligently cared for after birth, it will grow up to be healthy. On the other hand, a child born of healthy parents that is improperly cared for will become ill and perhaps die young.

In early years the habits are formed that will largely influence and control the years of maturity. Most children learn bad habits from birth. It is as easy to acquire good habits as bad ones, and as people are largely creatures of habits, every parent should aim to give his children a good start. Parents seldom do wrong intentionally, but they are careless and many of the parental habits of the race are bad, and for this the future generations must suffer.

It is easier and more economical to have healthy babies than to have sickly ones. The healthy way is the simple way. It merely means self-control, common sense and constructive knowledge on the part of the parents.

PRENATAL CARE.

It is commonly believed that a pregnant woman must eat for two. The wise woman will not increase her food intake. If she is not up to par physically at the time of conception she will generally find it advantageous to decrease the food allowance.

A healthy baby should not weigh to exceed six, or at most seven, pounds at birth. Five pounds would be better. It does not take much food to nourish an infant of that weight, and the baby does not weigh that much until shortly before birth. Most of the food is used for fuel but the amount of fuel required to heat a baby that is kept warm within the mother's body is almost negligible.

One of the first and most important requisites for having healthy children is to avoid the eating-for-two fallacy. Most people overeat, anyway, and there should be no encouragement in this line.

The results of overeating are many and serious. The mother grows too heavy or else she becomes dyspeptic. Overeating and partaking of food of poor quality are the chief causes of the ills of pregnancy. Prospective mothers can be comfortable. Pregnancy and childbirth are physiological. Normal women suffer very little inconvenience or pain. The suffering during pregnancy, the pain and accidents at childbirth are measures of the mother's abnormality. The greater the inconvenience the farther has the individual strayed from a natural life. The women who live normally from the time of conception, or before, until the birth of the baby will be surprised how little inconvenience there is.

For ideal results the father must be kind, considerate and self-controlled. It is a disagreeable fact that many men are brutal and inconsiderate of wives and unborn children. The extent of this brutality can hardly be realized by those who have had no medical experience. Perhaps the women are partly to blame, for they do not teach their boys to be considerate and kind and they leave them in ignorance of subjects that are important and that can best be taught by parents.

A pregnant woman should be mistress of her body. During this period the husband has morally no marital rights. If boys were educated by their parents on this subject they would be reasonable later on, and the average boy of fourteen or fifteen is old enough to receive such education.

Gestation should be a period of calm. All excitement and passion are harmful. The mother should be as free from annoyance as possible. Cheerfulness should be the rule. Those who are not naturally cheerful should cultivate this desirable state of mind. Gruesome and horrible topics should not be discussed. The reading should not be along tragic lines. The study of nature and the philosophy of men who have found life sweet are among the helpful mental occupations. The mental attitude has its effect, not only on the mother, but on the unborn babe. That the seed for good or evil is often planted in the child's brain before birth, according to the mental and physical condition of the mother, can hardly be doubted. Mothers who live naturally can dismiss all worry on the subject of harm coming to themselves through maternity, for there will be none. The absence of worry has a good effect on both mother and child.

The various ills from which mothers suffer are largely caused by eating for two. The overeating causes overweight in those whose nutrition is above par and indigestion in those who have but ordinary digestive capacity. Those who are overweight have too high blood pressure and those who have indigestion absorb some of the poisonous products of decomposition from the bowels. Headache is a common result. Palpitation of the heart comes from gas pressure. The abnormal blood pressure may result in albuminurea, swelling of the lower extremities and overweight of both mother and child. The morning sickness is nearly always due to excessive food intake. If this proves troublesome, reduce the amount of food and simplify the combinations. Instead of taking heavy, rich dishes, increase the amount of fresh fruits and vegetables.

The birth of a large baby is fraught with danger to mother and child. Sometimes one or both are injured and sometimes one or both die. Many women are afraid to become mothers for this reason. It would be difficult to estimate how often this fear causes law breaking, for all large cities have their medical men who grow rich through illegal practices among these women. Sometimes these doctors are among the respected members of the profession, eminent enough to have a national reputation. The financial reward is great enough to tempt men to break the law and they will continue to do so, so long as present conditions exist.

It is important for the prospective mother to be moderate in her eating. Three meals a day are sufficient. Between meals nothing but water should be swallowed. Lunching always leads to overeating.

One meal each day can consist of starchy food, but not more than one meal. Any one of the starches may be selected, the cereal products, rice, potatoes, chestnuts. If the digestion is good, take matured beans, peas or lentils occasionally, but these are so heavy that they should not be eaten very frequently and always in moderation. With the starchy food selected, take either butter or milk, or a moderate quantity of both. Sometimes it is all right to take some fruit with the starchy food, but this should be the exception, not the rule. Fruit should generally be eaten by itself or taken with non-starchy foods. Starch eating should be limited to one meal a day because an excessive amount of this food causes hardening of the tissues. The baby's bones, which should be very soft, flexible and yielding at birth, will become too hard if much starch is eaten.

Once a day some kind of proteid food may be taken, but this should also be eaten in moderation, for if it is not, degenerative changes will take place, which will manifest in some one of the disorders common to pregnancy. Eggs and the lighter kinds of meats, or nuts or fresh fish may be selected. Whatever kind of protein is taken, it should be as fresh as possible. Pork should not be used. With the protein, have either fruit or vegetables, and it does not make much difference which. No one could ask for a better meal than good apples and pecans.

Be sure to eat enough of the raw salad vegetables and of raw fruits to supply the salts needed by the body.

For the third meal have fruit. Cottage cheese, sweet or clabbered milk or buttermilk may be taken with the fruit. Do not take milk twice a day, for if it is taken twice and other proteid food once a day, too much protein is ingested.

A glass or two of buttermilk will make a good meal at any time. Dr. Waugh, who has had over forty years of experience and is well and favorably known on both sides of the Atlantic, recommends buttermilk very highly during pregnancy. Buttermilk and clabbered milk are better than the sweet milk. The lactic acid seems to have a sweetening effect on the alimentary tract. Sweet milk is constipating for many people. The buttermilk and the clabbered milk are not constipating to the same degree.

The use of fruit and vegetables has a tendency to prevent constipation. The only internal remedies for which there is any excuse are cathartics, and normal people do not need them. However, it is better to take a mild cathartic or an enema than to allow the colon to become loaded with waste. Constipation among eaters of much meat is rather a serious condition, for the waste in the colon of heavy meat eaters is very poisonous. The colonic waste in vegetarians is not so toxic.

Desserts should be used sparingly and seldom. They are not a necessity, but a habit, and if they are consumed daily they are a bad habit.

For the sake of the unborn child, avoid all stimulants and narcotics.

Alcoholics and coffee should not be used. And it is best to avoid strong spices and rich gravies. A little self-denial and self-control in this line will pay great dividends in healthy, happy, contented babies, and there are no greater blessings.

The mother should be active, but should not take any violent exercise. Light work is good, but no mother should Be asked to do house-cleaning or to stand over the wash-tub. She should have the opportunity of being in the open every day, and of this opportunity she should avail herself. Why some women are ashamed of pregnancy is hard for normal-minded people to understand, for the praise of motherhood has been sung by the greatest poets and its glory depicted by the greatest painters of the world.

This sense of false modesty is responsible for much of the tight lacing during pregnancy. This is injurious to both the mother and the child, and is one of the reasons for various uncomfortable sensations. It helps to bring on the morning sickness. It is nature's intention that the young should be free and comfortable previous to birth, and for this reason a double bag is supplied between the walls of which there is fluid. The baby lies within the inner bag.

The tight lacing prevents the intended freedom, besides weakening the mother's muscles. It also aggravates any tendency there may be toward constipation and swelling of the legs. It prolongs childbirth and makes it more painful. This is too high a price to pay for false modesty and vanity.

If it is necessary to support the abdomen and the breasts for the sake of comfort, this can be done without compressing them and the support should come from the shoulders.

The skin should be given good attention, for an active skin helps to keep the blood pure and the circulation normal. Take a vigorous dry rubbing at least once a day, and twice a day would be better. A quick sponging off with cool water followed with vigorous dry rubbing is good, but the rubbing is of greater importance than the sponging. An olive oil rub is often soothing and may be taken as frequently as desired.

If there is a tendency to be ill and nervous, take a good hot bath, staying in the water until there is a feeling of ease, even if it should take more than thirty minutes, provided the heart and the kidneys are working well. Defective heart and kidney action contraindicate prolonged hot baths, but such ills will not appear if the mother lives properly. Under such conditions missing a few meals can only have good results. When eating is resumed, partake of only enough food to nourish the body, for anything beyond that builds discomfort and disease.

These hints, simple as they are, contain enough information to rob gestation and childbirth of their horrors, if they are intelligently observed. If civilized woman desires to be as painfree as the savage, she must lead the simple life.

INFANCY.

If the baby lives to be one year old, its chances of surviving are fairly good, but during the first year the mortality is appalling. Complete statistics are not available, but in places one-fifth or even one-fourth of the babies born perish during this time. The mortality is chiefly due to overfeeding and giving food of poor quality.

The average parent loves his baby. He loves the helpless little thing to death. In Oscar Wilde's words, "We kill the thing we love." The babies are killed by too much love, which takes the form of overindulgence. About thirty years ago the well known physician, Charles B. Page, wrote:

"How many healthy-born infants die before their first year is reached--babies that for months are mistakenly regarded as pictures of health--'never knew a sick day until they were attacked' with cholera infantum, scarletina, or something else. They are crammed with food, made gross with fat, and for a time are active and cunning, the delight of parents and friends--and then, after a season of constipation, a season of chronic vomiting, and a season of cholera infantum, the little emaciated skeletons are buried in the ground away from the sight of those who have literally loved them to death. This is the fate of one-third of all the children born. As a rule, babies are fed as an ignorant servant feeds the cook-stove--filling the fire-box so full, often, that the covers are raised, the stove smokes and gases at every hole, and the fire is either put out altogether, or, if there is combustion of the whole body of coals, the stove is rapidly burned out and destroyed. With baby, overheating means the fever that consumes him, and, in putting out the fire, too often the fire of life goes out also."

Fat babies are thought to be healthy babies. This is a mistake, for the fatter the baby, the more liable it is to fill an early grave. Thoughtful, knowing people realize that a child that weighs eight pounds or more at birth is an indication of maternal law breaking. Both the mother and the child will have to pay for this sooner or later. Overweight is a handicap. It prevents complete internal cleansing and combustion, without which health is impossible.

Because of the false ideas prevalent regarding weight of infants, it is well to put a little emphasis on the subject. If the mother has lived right during pregnancy, the child is often light at birth, sometimes five pounds or less. The average doctor will shake his head and say that the baby's chance to live is very small. The friends, neighbors and relatives will say the same. They are wrong. Let the parents remember that light children are not encumbered with fat, and rarely with disease. A light baby is generally all healthy baby, and if properly cared for and not overfed will thrive. Parents of such babies should be thankful, instead of being alarmed.

It is not natural for babies to weigh nine or ten pounds at birth, and when they do it is a sign of maternal wrong doing, whether she has been cognizant of it or not. Babies should not be fat, nor should they be fat when they grow older, if the best results are desired.

In babies it is better to strive for quality than for quantity.

Every mother who is capable of doing so should nurse her baby. There is no food to take the place of the mother's milk. The babies build greater strength and resistance when they are fed naturally than when they are brought up on the bottle. Babies thrive wonderfully in an atmosphere of love, and they draw love from the mother's breast with every swallow.

From the information available, which is not as complete and definite as could be desired, it appears that from six to thirteen bottle-babies die during the first year where only one breast-fed child perishes. The bottle-baby does not get a fair start. If a mother is ill and worn out she should not be asked to nurse the baby. If the mother has fever she should not risk the baby's health through nursing. Some mothers do not have enough milk to feed the baby.

Nearly all who live properly give enough milk to nourish their infants at first. If there is not enough milk, the child should be allowed to take what there is in the breasts and this should be supplemented with cow's milk.

Dr. Thomas F. Harrington said recently:

"From 80 to 90 per cent. of all deaths from gastrointestinal disease among infants takes place in the artificially fed; or ten bottle-babies die to one which is breast-fed. In institutions it has been found that the death rate is frequently from 90 to 100 per cent. when babies are separated from their mothers. During the siege of Paris (1870-71) the women were compelled to nurse their own babies on account of the absence of cow's milk. Infant mortality under one year fell from 33 to 7 per cent. During the cotton famine of 1860 women were not at work in the mills. They nursed their babies and one-half of the infant mortality disappeared."

These are remarkable facts and bring home at least two truths. First, they confirm the superiority of natural feeding over that of artificial feeding. Second, they show that when the mother is not overfed the infants are healthier. During the siege of Paris food was scarce in that city. People of all classes had to live quite frugally. They could not overeat as in the untroubled time of peace and prosperity, and the result was that both the mothers and the babies were healthier. The infant mortality was only a little over one-fifth of what it was previously. If the French people had heeded the lesson the statesmen and philosophers of that nation would not today have to worry about its almost stationary population.

It would be much better if fewer children were born and those few were healthier. What good does the birth of the army of 425,000 children which perishes annually accomplish? It leaves the nation poorer in every way. A mother tired and worn with wakeful vigils, and at last left with an aching heart through the loss of her child, is not worth as much as she who has a crooning infant to love, and through her mother-love radiates kindness and good cheer to others. The conditions that weed out so many of our infants tend to weaken the survivors.

It costs too much to bring children into the world to waste them so lavishly. This may sound peculiar, but it is enlightened selfishness, which is the highest good, for it brings blessings upon all.

Artificial feeding lays the foundation for many troubles which may not manifest for several years. The bottle-fed babies are often plump, even fat, but they are not as strong as those who are fed naturally. They take all kinds of children's diseases very quickly. The glandular system, which is so readily disturbed in children, is more easily affected in bottle-fed babies. And so it comes about that they often have swollen salivary glands, or swelling of the glands of the neck or of the tonsils.

Do not be in a hurry to feed the baby after birth. Nature has so arranged that the infant does not require immediate feeding. It is a good plan to wait at least twenty-four hours after birth before placing the baby at the breast, for then all the tumult and excitement have had a chance to subside.

Many give the baby a cathartic within a few hours after birth. This is a mistake. Cathartics are irritants and it is a very poor beginning to abuse the mucous membrane of the intestinal tract immediately. This mucous membrane is delicate and in children the digestive apparatus is easily upset. Before birth there was no stomach or bowel digestion, all the nutritive processes taking place in the tissues of the little body. Gentle treatment is necessary to bring the best results. Cathartics with their harsh action on the delicate membranes are contraindicated. The mother's first milk is cathartic enough to stimulate the bowels to act, but it is nature's cathartic and does no harm.

As a rule the baby is fed too often and too much from the time of birth. If the child appears healthy the physician's recommendation will probably be to feed every two hours day and night, or every two hours during the day and every three hours at night. If the little one appears weakly these feedings are increased in number. From ten to twenty-four feedings in twenty-four hours are not uncommon and sometimes infants are nursed or given the bottle two and even three times an hour. The excuse for this is that the baby's stomach is small and cannot hold much food at a time and must for this reason be filled often, for the baby has to grow, and the more food it gets the faster it grows. The baby's stomach is small, because the little one needs very little food. The human being grows and develops for twenty to twenty-five years. This growth is slow and during babyhood the amount of nourishment needed is not great. The child, if properly taken care of, is kept warm. Hence it needs but little fuel. The ideas on food needs are so exaggerated that it is hard for parents to realize what moderate amount of food will keep a baby well nourished.

An adult in the best of health would be unable to stand such frequent food intake. He would be ill in a short time. Babies stand it no better, and the only proof of this fact needed is that in the United States at least 280,000 babies under one year of age perish annually. During babyhood nearly all troubles are nutritive ones. With the stomach and bowels in excellent condition baby defies all kinds of diseases, provided it is given the simple, commonsense attentions needed otherwise, such as being kept warm and clean in a well ventilated room. With a healthy alimentary canal, which comes with proper feeding, the little one can withstand the attack of the vast horde of germs which so trouble adult minds, also adult bodies, when people fail to give themselves proper care.

The results of too frequent feeding and overfeeding are appalling. The first ill effect is digestive disturbance. Then one or more of the ills of childhood make their appearance. These are called diseases, but they are only symptoms of perverted nutrition, though we insist on giving them names.

A healthy baby is one that is absolutely normal and well in every way. However, babies today pass for healthy when they are fat and suffering from all kinds of troubles, provided these ills can be tolerated. We need a new standard of health. Perfect health is a gift that every normal parent can bestow upon his children, and we should be satisfied with nothing short of this. Babies can and should be raised without illness, but, sad to relate, babies, who are always healthy are so rare that they are curiosities.

Many babies show signs of maternal overfeeding within a few hours or days of birth. One of the common signs is the discharge from the nose. This is aggravated by overfeeding the infant. And thus is laid the foundation, perhaps, for a lifelong catarrh. In due time various diseases such as rickets, swollen glands, formerly called scrofulous, mumps, measles, scarlet fever, diphtheria, pimples, eczema and cholera infantum, make their appearance. Parents have been taught to look for these diseases. They have been told that they belong to childhood. This is a libel on nature, for she tends in the direction of health.

The prevalent idea at present is that various germs, which are found in water, food, air and earth, are responsible for these diseases, but they are not. The fact that infants properly cared for do not develop one of them is proof enough that germs per se are unable to cause these ills. The germs play their part in most of these diseases, but it is a kindly part. They are scavengers, and attempt to rid the body of its debris and poisons. Through false reasoning they are blamed for causing disease, when in fact their multiplication is an effect. They are a by-product of disease. The so-called pathogenic bacteria never thrive in the baby's body until the infant has been overfed or fed on improper food long enough to break down its resistance.

The improper feeding not only kills an army of babies each year, but it handicaps the survivors very seriously. The degenerated condition of the system leaves every child with some kind of weakness. The foundation may be laid for indigestion, catarrhal troubles, which may or may not be accompanied with adenoids and impeded breathing, glandular troubles, often precursors of tuberculosis, in fact children may be acquiring any disease during infancy from chronic catarrh to rheumatism.

Mental ills are also results of senseless feeding. A healthy baby is happy. A sick baby is cross. Crossness and anger are mental perversions. Anger is temporary insanity. Enough overfeeding often results in mental perversity, epilepsy and even in real insanity. A healthy body gives a healthy mind. If people would care for their bodies properly, especially in the line of eating, the asylums for the insane would not be needed for their present purposes.

Another serious trouble that takes root from infant overfeeding is an abnormal craving for stimulants. This craving may later on be satisfied in many ways. Some use coffee, alcohol, habit-forming drugs. Others try to satisfy it by overeating. No matter how the sufferer proceeds to satisfy this craving, he does not cure it, for it grows upon what it is fed. Morphine calls for more morphine. Tobacco calls for more tobacco. An oversupply of food calls for more food or alcohol. The victim at last dies a martyr to his abnormal appetites.

Comparatively few of those who see the error of their ways have the will power to thrust off the shackles of habit. Very few think clearly enough and go far enough back to realize that disease and early death are so largely due to the habits formed for the infant or unborn babe by the parents. And the parents received the same kind of undesirable legacy from their parents, and so it goes, the children suffering for the sins of the parents. The cheerful part of such a retrospect is that there is much room for improvement, that we need not continue this seemingly unending chain of physical bondage to the next generation, and that if the children are not born right or treated right during infancy, there is still time to make a change for the better. Nature is kind and with will and determination a change can be made at any time that will result in betterment, provided such grave diseases have not taken hold of the body that recuperation is impossible. This is no excuse for making delays, for the longer errors are permitted the harder they are to overcome.

Three or four feedings a day are sufficient for any baby. The feedings should be arranged so that they are evenly distributed during the day, and nothing is to be given at night except water. Get a nursing bottle or two. Keep the bottles and the nipples scrupulously clean. These are to be used as water bottles. The water must also be clean. Heat it to 103 or 104 degrees Fahrenheit, so that it will be from 98 to 100 degrees warm when it enters the baby's mouth Let the baby have some water three or four times during the day, and perhaps it will want some once or twice during the night, but give it no milk at night.

Overfed babies are irritable and cry often. The mothers interpret this as a sign of hunger. Most babies do not know what hunger is. Like adults they become thirsty, but instead of getting water to quench their thirst they are given milk. This satisfies for a little while, then the irritability due to milk spoiled, in the alimentary tract causes more restlessness and crying, and they are fed again. The comedy of errors continues until it is turned into a tragedy.

How much should the baby be fed at a time? When the parents are healthy and the baby is born right and then fed but three times a day, the food intake will regulate itself. The child will not usually want more than it should have of milk, supplemented with water. The best way to begin is to let the infant take what it desires. That is, let the nursing continue while the infant manifests great pleasure and zest. When the child begins to fool with the breast or bottle, the source of nourishment should be removed immediately. The child will increase its intake gradually.

Some of the babies will take too much. The evil results will soon be evident, and then the mother must not compromise, but reduce the intake at once. The signs of over-consumption of food by the infants are the same as those shown by adults. They are discomfort and disease. The former manifests in crossness and irritability. The disease may be of any kind, ranging from a rash to a high fever.

The baby's stomach is sensitive and resents the excessive amount of food supplied. So the infant often vomits curdled milk, and some times vomits before the milk has time to curdle. This is a form of self-protection. If the mother would heed this sign by withdrawing all food until the stomach is settled, substituting water in the meanwhile, and then reduce the baby's food to within digestive capacity, there would be no more trouble. Vomiting is the infant's way of saying, "Please do not feed me until my stomach becomes normal again, and then don't give me more than I need, and that is less than I have been getting." Remember that it is nature's sign language, which never misleads, and it is so plain that any one with ordinary understanding should get its meaning, in spite of the erroneous popular teachings. After the child has vomited, feed moderately and increase its food supply as its digestive ability increases.

If the vomiting is wrongly interpreted and overfeeding is continued, either the baby dies or the stomach establishes a toleration, passing the trouble on to other parts of the body. One organ never suffers long alone. The circulation passes the disease on to other parts, assisted by the sympathetic nerves, which are present in all parts of the body.

When the stomach has established its toleration, several things may happen, only a few of which will be discussed, for the process is essentially the same, though the results appear so different. In infants whose digestive power is not very strong the excessive amount of milk curdles, as does the part that is digested. The water of the milk is absorbed, but the curds pass into the colon without being digested and they are discharged in the stool as curds. They are partly decomposed on the journey through the alimentary canal, producing poisons, a part of which is absorbed. A part remains in the colon, making the bowel discharges very offensive.

The passage of curds in the stool is a danger signal indicating overfeeding and should be heeded immediately. If it is not, the chances for a ease of cholera infantum, especially in warm weather, are great. Cholera infantum is due to overfeeding, or the use of inferior milk, or both. It is a form of milk poisoning, in which the bowels are very irritable. As a matter of self-protection they throw out a large quantity of serum, which soon depletes the system of the poor little sufferer, and death too often claims another young life. If cholera infantum makes its appearance the baby is given its best chance to live if feeding is stopped immediately, warm water given whenever desired, but not too large quantities at a time. Give no cathartics, for they irritate an already seriously disturbed mucous membrane, but give a small enema of blood-warm water once or twice a day. Keep the baby comfortable, seeing that the feet and abdomen are kept warm, but give plenty of fresh air. Medicines only aggravate a malady that is already serious enough. This disease is produced by abuse so grave that in spite of the best nursing, the baby often dies. It is easily prevented.

Strong babies with great digestive power are often able to digest and assimilate enormous quantities of milk, several quarts a day. They can not use all this food. If they could their size would be enormous within a short time. They do not find it so easy to excrete the excess as to assimilate it. The skin, kidneys, lungs and the bowels find themselves overtaxed. Often the mucous membrane of the nose and throat are called upon to assist in the elimination. These are the babies who are said to catch cold easily. Their colds are not caught. They are fed to them. This constant abuse of the mucous membrane results in inflammation, subacute in nature, or it may be so mild that it is but an irritation. The result in time may be chronic catarrh or thickening of the mucous membrane of nose and throat. While the catarrh is being firmly established adenoids are quite common.

In other cases too much of the work of excretion is thrown upon the skin. The same thing happens to this structure as happens to the mucous membrane. It is made for a limited amount of excretion and when more foreign matter, much of it of a very irritating nature, is deposited for elimination through the skin, it becomes inflamed. It itches. In a little while there is an attack of eczema. The baby scratches, digging its little nails in with a will. The infant soon has its face covered with sores and the scalp is scaly.

The proper thing to do is to reduce the feeding greatly. Then the acid-producing fermentation in stomach and bowels will cease, but enough food to nourish the body will be absorbed, the skin will have but its normal work to perform, the cause of the irritation is gone and the effects will disappear in a short time. Two weeks are often sufficient to bring back the smooth, soft skin that every baby should have. The sufferers from these troubles are almost invariably overweight, and the parents wonder why their babies, who are so healthy, should be troubled thus!

Mothers owe it to their nursing babies to lead wholesome, simple lives. It is not always possible to live ideally, but every mother can eat simply and control her temper. Wholesome food and equanimity will go far toward producing healthful nourishment for the child. Stimulants and narcotics should be avoided. Meat should not be eaten more than once a day, and it would be better to use less meat and more eggs or nuts. Fresh fruits and vegetables should be partaken of daily. They are the rejuvenators and purifiers. The cereal foods should be as near natural as possible. The bread should be made of whole wheat flour mostly. If rice is eaten it should be unpolished. Refined sugar should be taken in moderation, if at all. The potatoes are best baked. Pure milk is as good for the mother as it is for the child. Highly seasoned foods or rich made dishes should be avoided. In short, the mother should live as near naturally as possible.

The importance of cheerfulness can hardly be overestimated. A nervous mother who frets or worries, or becomes mastered by any of the negative, depressing passions, poisons her babe a little with each drop of milk the child takes.

Some mothers are unable to nurse their babies. This is so because of lack of knowledge principally, for women who give themselves proper care are nearly always able to furnish nourishment for their infants. It may be that this function will be largely lost if the present preponderance of artificial feeding continues, and if various inoculations are not stopped. Some mothers find it a great pleasure to nurse their babies. Others refuse to do so for fear of ruining their figures.

No matter what the reason is for depriving the infant of its natural food, the parents should realize that its chances for health and life are diminished by this act. If intelligence and care are used in raising the bottle-fed babies only a few will die, in fact none will die under the circumstances, provided they were born with a normal amount of resistance. So it behooves parents of such babies to be extremely careful. That there are difficulties in the way, or rather inconveniences, can not be denied, but there are no insurmountable obstacles.

The best common substitute for mother's milk is cow's milk. If clean and given in moderation it will agree with the child and produce no untoward results.

Instead of using the same bottle all the time, there should be a number, so that there will be plenty of time to clean them. If three feeds are given each day, there should be six bottles. If four feeds are given, eight bottles. Use a set every other day. The bottles should be rinsed out after being used. Then boil them in water containing soda or a little lye, rinse in several waters and set them aside. If it is sunny, let them stand in the sun. Before using, rinse again in sterile water. The nipples should have equally good care. In feeding babies cleanliness comes before godliness.

Each bottle is to be used for but one feeding, and as many bottles are to be prepared as there are to be feedings for the day.

If the people live in the country it is easy to get pure milk. If in the city one should make arrangements with a reliable milk man possessed of a conscience. It is well to get the milk from a certain cow, instead of taking a mixture coming from many cows. Select a healthy animal that does not give very rich milk, such as the Holstein. She should have what green food she wants every day, grass in summer, and hay of the best quality and silage in winter. The grain ration should be moderate, for cows that are forced undergo quick degeneration. They are burned out. The cow should not be worried or whipped. She should be allowed to be happy, and animals are happy if they are treated properly. The water supply should be clean, not from one of the filthy tubs or troughs which disgrace some farms. The barn should be light and well ventilated. It should be kept clean and free from the ammonia fumes which are found in filthy stables. The cow should be brushed and the udder washed before each milking. The milker should wash his hands and have on clothes from which no impurities will fall. The first part of the milk drawn should not be put in with that which is to supply the baby. The milk should be drawn into a clean receptacle and immediately strained through sterile surgeon's cotton into glass bottles. These are to be put aside to cool, the contents not exposed to the dust falling from the air. Or the milk may be put directly into the nursing bottles and put aside in a cold place until needed. Then warm milk to 100 degrees Fahrenheit.

Pardon a little repetition: If possible let the child nurse. If there is not enough milk, let the baby take what there is and give cow's milk in addition. If it is impossible to feed the baby at the breast, get the milk from a healthy cow that is kept clean, well fed and well treated. The cow's milk should be prepared as follows: Take equal parts of milk and water. Or take two parts of milk and one part of water. Mix, and to this may be added sugar of milk in the proportion of one level teaspoonful to the quart. Before feeding raise the temperature of the milk to about 104 degrees Fahrenheit, so that it will be about 100 degrees when fed. It is best to do the warming in a water bath.

Milk should not be kept long before being used. Limit the age to thirty-six hours after being drawn from the cow. Twenty-four hours would be better. The evening milk can safely be given to the infant the next day, if proper precautions have been taken. Ordinary milk is quite filthy and upon this babies do not thrive. Make an effort to get clean milk for the baby.

The composition of human milk and cow's milk is about as follows:

```
===============================================================
===== Water Albumin Fat Sugar Salts --------------------------------------------------
--------------- Human .......... 87.58 2.01 3.74 6.37 .30 Cow's .......... 87.27 3.39
3.68 4.97 .72 -----------------------------------------------------------------------
```

The albumin in human milk is largely of a kind which is not coagulated by souring, while nearly all the albumin in cow's milk coagulates. The uncoagulated albumin is digested and taken up more easily by the baby's nutritive system than that which is coagulated. This is one of the reasons that babies do not thrive so well on cow's milk as on their natural food.

The sugar of milk is not like refined sugar. Although it is not so easily dissolved in water, and therefore does not taste as sweet as refined sugar, it is better for the child. If sugar is added to the milk, milk sugar should be used. The druggists have it in powder form.

The addition of barley water and lime to the baby's milk is folly. The various forms of modified milk do not give as good results as the addition of water and a little milk sugar, as previously described. If you believe in such modifications as the top milk method and the addition of starchy substances and lime water, I refer you to your family physician or text-books on infant feeding.

It is difficult to improve on good cow's milk. It is well to remember that the human organism is very adaptable, even in infancy. The principal factors in infant feeding are cleanliness and moderation.

Bottle-fed babies should be given fruit or vegetable juices, or both, very early and it would be well to give a little of these juices to breast-fed babies too. The latter do not require as much as the former. Begin during the first month with a teaspoonful of orange juice put into the drinking bottle once a day. Increase gradually until at four or five months the amount may be from one to two tablespoonfuls. Do not be afraid to give the orange juice because it is acid, for it splits up quickly in the stomach and is rearranged, forming alkaline salts. It is the fruit that can be obtained at nearly all seasons. It is best to get mild oranges and strain the juice. The fruit is to be in prime condition. Instead of orange juice, the juice of raw celery, spinach, cabbage, apples, blackberries and other juicy fruits and vegetables may be employed, but these juices must all come from fruits or vegetables that are in prime condition. No sugar is to be added to either the fruit or the vegetable juices.

The mother's milk coagulates in small flakes, easily acted upon by the digestive juices, after which they are readily absorbed. Cow's milk coagulates into rather large pieces of albumin which are tough and therefore rather difficult to digest. This happens when the milk is taken rapidly and undiluted. However, when diluted and taken slowly this tendency is overcome to a great degree. For this reason it is best to get nipples with small perforations.

Either pasteurization or sterilization of milk is almost universally recommended by medical men. Even those who do not believe in such procedures generally fail to condemn them without qualifying statements. For a discussion of this fallacy I refer you to the chapter on milk.

Do not give the little ones any kinds of medicines. They always do harm and never any good. If any exception is made to this, it is in the line of laxatives or mild cathartics, such as small doses of castor oil, cascara segrada or mineral waters, but there is no excuse for giving metallic remedies, such as calomel. If the babies are fed in moderation on good foods they will not become constipated. If they are imprudently handled and become constipated it is necessary to resort to either the enema or some mild cathartic. Bear in mind that such remedies do not cure. They only relieve. The cure will come when the errors of life are corrected so that the body is able to perform its work without being obstructed.

Inoculations and vaccinations are serious blunders, often fatal. The animal products that are rubbed or injected into the little body are poisonous. They are the result of degenerative changes--diseases--in the bodies of rabbits, horses, cows and other animals. Nature's law is that health must be deserved or earned. Health means cleanliness, so it really is absurd to force into the body these products of animal decay. Statistics can be given, showing how beneficial these agents are, but they are misleading. In the days of public and official belief in witchcraft it was not difficult to prove the undoubted existence of witches. Whatever the public accepts as true can with the utmost ease be bolstered up with figures.

The use of serums, bacterins, vaccines and other products of the biologic laboratory is almost an obsession today. Their curative and preventive values are taken for granted. Most of the time the children are strong enough to throw off the poisons without showing prolonged or pronounced effects, but every once in a while a child is so poisoned that it takes months for it to regain health and too often death is the end. Sometimes the death takes place a few minutes after the injection, but we are informed that the medication had nothing to do with it. To poison the baby's blood deliberately is criminal. Give the little one a fair chance to live in health. A properly cared for baby will not be ill for one single day. Knowledge and good care will prevent sickness.

A baby that is able to remain well a month or a week or a day can remain well every day.

At first a normal baby sleeps nearly all the time, from twenty to twenty-two hours a day. The infant should not be disturbed. All that should be done for it is to feed it three times a day, give it some water from the bottle three or four times a day, and keep it clean, dry and warm, but not hot.

Most babies are bathed daily. This is all right, but the baths are to be given quickly. The water should be about 100 degrees Fahrenheit. The soap should be of the mildest, such as a good grade of castile, and it should be well rinsed off, for soap permitted to remain in the pores acts as an irritant. Dry the skin so well with a soft cloth that there will be no chapping or roughness. Sores, eruptions and inflammations are signs of mismanagement. Use no powders that are metallic in character, such as zinc oxide. A dusting powder of finely ground talcum is good. If the child is kept dry and dean and moderately fed the skin will remain in good condition.

Babies do not thrive without good air. Keep the room well ventilated at all times by admitting fresh air from a source that will produce no draughts. It is not necessary to have the baby's room warm. In fact a cool room is better. When the child is to be exposed to the air, take it into a warm room. Soft coverings will keep the infant warm. The limbs should be free so that exercise can be had through unrestricted movements.

The baby should not be bothered unnecessarily. Young parents make the mistake of using the baby for show purposes. For the sake of politeness, others praise the "only baby in the world" unduly, though there are millions of others just as good. Let the child alone, thus giving it an opportunity to become as superior as the parents think it is. The showing off process creates excitement and lays the foundation for fretfulness, irritability and nervousness. The child thrives in a peaceful atmosphere. When it is awake it is well to talk to it quietly and soothingly, for thus the infant begins to learn its mother's tongue. Good language should be employed. Those who teach their children baby-talk are handicapping them, for they will soon have to unlearn this and learn real language. Baby-talk may be "cute" at eighteen months, but when children retain that mode of expression beyond the age of four or five it sounds silly.

At about the age of nine or ten months the breast-fed babe should be weaned. Gradual weaning is perhaps the best. First give one feeding of cow's milk a day and two breast feeds; then two feedings of cow's milk and one at the breast, and at last cow's milk entirely. Between the ages of nine and twelve months begin giving starchy foods. At first the child will take very little, and gradually increase. Give bread so stale that the child has to soak it with its saliva before it can swallow the bread. Working away this way, sucking the stale bread, the child learns to go through the motions of chewing, and this is valuable training. Never give bread soaked in milk and never feed milk while bread is being eaten. If the meal is to be bread and milk, give the bread either before any milk is taken, or afterwards. Starches are not to be washed down with liquids. Instead of giving stale bread, zwieback may be used. Occasionally feed a few spoons of very thin and well cooked oatmeal or whole wheat gruel, but the less sloppy food given the better, for it does not get the proper mouth treatment. The wheat products fed the child should be made from whole wheat flour, or at least three-fourths whole wheat and only one-fourth of the white flour. The refined flour is lacking in the salts that the child needs for health and growth.

Many mothers begin feeding starches when the baby is four or five months old. The child is given potatoes, bread or any other starchy food that may be on the table. This is a mistake, for the child is not prepared to digest starches at that early age. Some of the digestive ferments are practically absent during the first few months of life. Such feeding will invariably cause trouble. The baby should not be taken to the table.

It is quite generally believed that a baby should cry to exercise its lungs. A healthy, comfortable baby will do little or no crying, and it is not necessary. It is not difficult to give the little ones some exercise to fill their lungs. Babies can hang on to a finger or a thin rod tenaciously. Elevate the infant that does not cry thus a few times above the bed and let it hang for a few seconds each time. This throws the chest forward and exercises the lungs. What is more, this small amount of gymnastic work is thoroughly enjoyed. It helps to build strength and good temper. The crying helps to make the baby ill-tempered and fretful. A little crying now and then is all right, but much indicates discomfort, disease or a spoiled child. It would surprise most mothers how good babies are when they have a chance to be good.

After reading this, some are sure to ask how many ounces to feed the baby. I don't know. No one else knows. Different babies have different requirements. The key is given above. If the babies become ill it is nearly always due to overfeeding and poor food, so the proper thing to do is to reduce the food intake.

A healthy baby is a source of unending joy, while a sick one saps the mother's vitality. It is too bad that the art of efficient child culture is so little known.

CHILDHOOD.

Children may roughly be divided into two types, the robust and the more delicate or nervous ones. The robust children can stand almost all kinds of abuse with no apparent harm resulting, but the immunity is only apparent. The growing child naturally throws off disease influences easily and quickly, but if the handicap is too great the child loses out in the race.

The nervous type can not be abused with impunity, for the bodies of these delicately balanced children are easily disturbed. They must have more intelligent care than is usually bestowed upon the robust type. If the care is not forthcoming they become weak in body, with an unstable nervous system, or perish early.

Some parents complain because other people's children can do what their own can not and they wonder why. No time should be wasted in making such comparisons, for no two children are exactly alike, as no two leaves and not even two such apparently similar objects as grains of wheat are exactly alike. Therefore the care necessary varies somewhat, though it is basically the same.

If the nervous type is given proper care, good health will be the result. These children do not tolerate as much exposure or as much food as do the robust children. The important thing is to learn what they require and then see that there is no excess, and in this way allow the child to grow physically strong and mentally efficient.

The delicate children are perhaps more fortunate than the stronger ones, for they learn early in life that they have limitations. If they commit excesses the results are so disagreeable that they soon learn to be prudent. This prudence serves as protection so long as life lasts.

The robust children on the other hand soon learn that they are strong. They hear their parents boast about it. They get the idea that because they are strong they will always remain so, that nothing will do them any serious harm. By living up to this fallacy they undermine their constitutions. Parents should teach their children about the law of compensation as applied to health, that is, he has permanent health who deserves it, and no one else. The children will not always heed true teachings after they have left the parental influence, but the parents have at least done the best they could.

The robust children have their troubles, such as chicken-pox, mumps, fevers and measles, but these are thrown off so quickly and with so little inconvenience that they are soon forgotten. As a rule the parents do not realize that these diseases are due to faulty nutrition, and that faulty nutrition is caused by improper feeding. It is generally believed that children must have all the so-called children's diseases. Some mothers expose their infants to all of these that may happen to be in the neighborhood, hoping that the children will take them and be through with them.

Every time a child is sick it is a reflection on either the intelligence or the performance of the parents. It is natural for children to be perfectly well, and they will remain in that happy state if they are given the opportunity. If they are properly fed they will not take any of the children's diseases in spite of repeated exposure. There is not a disease germ known to medical science strong enough to establish itself in the system of an uninjured, healthy child and do damage. The child's health must first be impaired, through poor care, and then the so-called disease germs will find a hospitable dwelling place. If children are given natural food in normal quantities they are disease-proof. Feeding them on refined sugar and white flour products, pasteurized or sterilized milk, potatoes fried in grease pickled meats, and various other ruined foods breaks down their resistance and then they fall an easy prey to disease.

Some parents make the mistake of believing that they can feed their children improperly and ward off disease by vaccinations or inoculations of the products of disease taken from various animals. This is contrary to reason, common sense and nature and it is impossible. Any individual who is continually abused in any way, be he infant or adult, will deteriorate. If the disease is not the one that has been feared, it will be some other one.

The robust children generally develop into careless adults. That is why so many of them, in fact the vast majority, die before they are fifty years old, although they are equipped with constitutions that were intended to last over a century. They are shining marks for typhoid fever, Bright's disease, various forms of heart and liver troubles, rheumatism and pneumonia, all of which are largely caused by too hearty eating. These diseases often come without apparent warning. That is, the victims have thought themselves healthy. However, they have not known what real health is. They have been in a state of tolerable health, not suffering any very annoying aches or pains, but they have lacked the normal state of body which results in a clear, keen mind. As a rule there is enough indigestion present to cause gas in the bowels and a coated tongue. Enough food is generally eaten to produce excessive blood pressure.

The foundation for such a state of affairs is laid in childhood, yes, often before the child is born. It can readily be seen how important it is for parents to impart a little sound health information to the children. At least, they should teach them what health really is, which many people do not know.

When these strong people become sick it is often difficult, or even impossible, to do anything for them, for their habits are so gross and have gained such a mastery that the patients will not or can not change their ways.

The weaklings have a better chance to survive to old age, because many of them learn to be careful early in life. In reading the lives of eminent men who have lived long it is common to find that they were never strong.

At the age of one year the baby is generally weaned. The ordinary child needs the mother's milk no longer, for by this time the digestive power is great enough to cope with cow's milk and various starches. The most important problem now is how to feed the child. If no errors of importance are made it will enjoy uninterrupted growth and health. If the errors are many and serious there will surely be disease and too often the abuse is so great that death comes and ends the suffering.

Until the child reaches the age of two years the best foods are milk, whole wheat products and fruits. No other foods are necessary. The simpler the baby's food, and the more naturally and plainly prepared, the better. Adults who overeat until they suffer from jaded appetites, may think that they need great variety of food, but it is never necessary for infants or normal adults. Milk, whole wheat and fruits contain all the elements needed for growth and strength and health. By all means feed simply. Children are perfectly satisfied with bread and milk or simply one kind of fruit at a meal, if they are properly trained. The craving for a great variety of foods at each meal is due to parental mismanagement.

Children should not be fed more than three times a day. There should be no lunching. The children will get all that is good for them, all they need in three meals. Candy should not be given between meals, and fruit is to be looked upon as a food, not as a dainty to be consumed at all hours of the day. If they are not accustomed to lunching, there will be no craving for lunches. If children are used to four or five meals a day they want them and raise annoying objections when deprived of one or two of them. It is easy to get children into bad habits. We can not blame the average mother for giving her children lunches, for she knows no better and sees other mothers doing the same.

The children who do not get lunches thrive better than those who always have candy, fruit or bread and jam at their command. It is the same with adults. In the Dakotas and Minnesota are many Scandinavians and Germans. During the haying and harvest these people, who are naturally very strong, eat four and five times a day. The heat, the excessive amount of food and the great quantities of coffee consumed cause much sickness during and after the season of hard work and heroic eating. The so-called Americans in these communities are generally satisfied with three meals a day, and they are as well nourished and capable of working as those who eat much more.

Refined sugar made from cane and beets should be given to children sparingly. Refined sugar is the chemical which is largely responsible for the perversion of children's tastes. A normal taste is very desirable, for it protects the possessor. A perverted taste, on the contrary, leads him into trouble. Sugar is not a good food. It is an extract. It is easy to cultivate a desire for sugar, but to people who are not accustomed to it, concentrated sugar has an unpleasant taste.

The perversion of the sense of taste, generally begun with sugar, is made worse by the use of much salt, pepper and various condiments and spices. If the child is fed on unnatural food, highly seasoned, at the age of a few years its taste is so perverted that it does not know how most of the common foods really taste, and refuses to eat the best of them when the health-destroying concoctions to which it has been accustomed can be had.

It is natural for children to relish fruit, but some are so perverted in taste that they object to a meal of it if they can get pancakes or waffles with butter and syrup, mushes with sugar and cream, ham or bacon with fried potatoes, or fresh bread and meat with pickles. Many parents allow their children to live on this class of food to the exclusion of all natural foods. Children need a great deal of the natural salts, and when they live so largely on denatured foods there is always physical deterioration. It is true that to the average eye such children may appear healthy, but they are not in one-half as good physical condition as they could be.

Tea and coffee should never be given to children. They are bad enough for adults. In children they retard bodily development. The stimulation and sedation are bad for the nervous system. Coffee is as harmful as tobacco for the growing child.

To warn against alcohol may seem foolish, but some parents really give beer and whiskey to their infants. The beer is given as a beverage and the whiskey as medicine to kill pain and soothe the children. Those who have not seen children abused in this way may find it difficult to believe that there is such a profundity of ignorance. These children die easily.

Others quiet their children with the various soothing syrups. The last analyses that came under my eyes showed that these remedies contained considerable opium, laudanum, morphine and other deadly poisons. Morphine and opium are not well borne by children and these "mother's friends" have soothed many a baby into the sleep from which there is no waking. Make it a rule to give the children no medicines, either patent or those prescribed by physicians. Please remember that any remedy that quiets a child is poisonous. Children who get proper care require no medical quieting.

Condiments should not be used. Salt is not necessary despite the popular belief to the contrary, though a small amount does no harm. Salt eating is a habit and when carried to excess it is a bad one. Salt is a good preservative, but there is little excuse for our using preserved foods extensively. There are so many foods that can be had without being preserved in this country that it would not be difficult to exclude these inferior foods from the dietary. Children whose foods are not seasoned do not desire seasoning, provided they are fed on natural foods from the start. They want the seasoning because they are taught to eat their food that way. If they are given fresh fruit every day, such as apples, oranges, cherries, grapes and berries, they get all the seasoning they need and they get it in natural form.

The objection is made that such feeding deprives children of many of the good things of life. This is not true. Natural foods taste better than the doctored ones every time. Nature imparts a flavor to food products which man has never been able to equal, to say nothing of surpassing it. Children are taught to like abnormal foods. What is better, to give children good foods upon which they thrive, or denatured foods which taste well to a perverted palate, but are injurious?

Instead of giving sugar or candy, give raisins, figs, dates or sweet prunes. Small children may be given the strained juices of these fruits, obtained either by soaking the raw fruits several hours or by stewing them. Children who are given these fruits do not crave refined sugar. They like these natural sugars better than the artificial extract. These sweet fruits take the place of starchy food.

Very few people know anything definite about food values. Those who have studied foods and their values in order to be able to feed children properly generally make the mistake of believing that they should have all the necessary elements at each meal in about the proper proportion. This is a grave mistake and leads to trouble. The child needs salts, protein, sugar and fat, and in the absence of sugar some starch. Milk contains all these substances except starch. Give one fruit meal and two meals of starch daily. Milk may be given with all the meals or it may be given but once or twice. Do not overfeed on milk, for it is a rich food.

Until the child is two years old, confine it in its starch eating pretty much to the products of whole wheat. Give no white bread. White bread is an unsatisfying form of food. It is so tasteless and insipid and so deprived of the natural wheat salts that too much has to be eaten to satisfy. Children who would be satisfied with a reasonable amount of whole wheat bread eat more white bread and still do not feel satisfied. The same is true of rice, the natural brown rice being so superior to the polished article that there is no comparison.

The bread should be toasted in the oven until it is crisp clear through, or else it should be stale. Let the bread for toast get stale, and then place it in the oven when this is cooling off. Make the slices moderately thin. This is an easy and satisfactory way of making toast. Scorched bread--what is usually called toast--is not fit food for young children.

After the second year is completed gradually increase the variety of starch. Some of the better forms of starch that are easy to obtain are: Puffed rice or puffed wheat; brown, unpolished rice; triscuit or shredded wheat biscuit; the prepared corn and wheat flakes; baked potatoes; occasionally well cooked oatmeal or whole wheatmeal gruel. Mushes are to be given seldom or never. Children seldom chew them well, and they require thorough mastication. The rice is not to be sugared but after the child has had enough, milk may be given. A small amount of butter may be served with either rice or baked potato. The cereal foods should be eaten dry. Let the children masticate them, as they should, and as they will not if the starches are moistened with milk. When they have had sufficient of these starches, and but one kind is to be served at a meal, give milk, if milk is to be a part of the meal. To observe the suggestions here given for the manner of feeding starches to children may mean the difference between success and failure in raising them. It is the little things that are important in the care of children.

The acid fruits should not be given in the meals containing starchy foods. Strong children who have plenty of opportunity to be in the fresh air and who are very active can stand this combination, but it is injurious to the nervous type. It is not a good thing to make such combinations habitually for robust children. A good meal can be made of fruit followed by milk. Do not slice the fruit, sprinkle it with sugar and cover it with cream. Give the child the fruit and nothing else. Neither oranges nor grapefruits are to be sugared. Their flavor is better without. If the children want sweets, give them a meal of sweet fruits.

When the child is eighteen months old it should have learned to masticate well enough to eat various fruits. Apples, oranges, grapefruits, berries, cherries, grapes and melons are among the foods that may be given. If the child does not masticate well, either grind the fruit or scrape it very fine. The sweet fruits require so much mastication that only their juices should be fed until the child is old enough to masticate thoroughly. Bananas should also be withheld until there is no doubt about the mastication. They must be thoroughly ripe, the skin being dark in spots and the flesh firm and sweet. A green banana is very starchy, but a ripe one contains hardly any starch and digests easily.

At first the meal is fruit, followed with milk. Buttermilk or clabbered milk may be substituted for sweet milk. A little later, begin giving cottage cheese occasionally in place of milk, if the child likes it.

The succulent vegetables may be given quite early. At the age of two years stewed onions, green peas, cauliflower, egg plant and summer squash may be given. Gradually increase the variety until all the succulent vegetables are used. At first it may be necessary to mash these vegetables.

The longer children go without meat the better, and if they never acquired the meat-eating habit it would be a blessing. If the parents believe in feeding their children meat, they should wait until the little ones are at least four years old before beginning. Meats are digestible enough, but too stimulating for young people. Chicken and other fowls may be used at first, and it is best to use young birds. Beef and pork should not be on the children's menu. At the age of seven or eight the variety may be increased. However, parents who wish to do the best by their children will give them little or no meat. Many of the sorrows that parents suffer through their wayward children would be done away with if the young people were fed on less stimulating foods.

Eggs are better for children than meat. However, it is not necessary to give them. The children get enough milk to supply all the protein they need. Eggs may be given earlier than meat. At the age of two and one-half years an egg may be given occasionally. At three they may be given every other day, one egg at a meal. At five or six years of age, an egg may be given daily, but not more than one at a time. If they are soft boiled, three and one-half minutes will suffice. If hard boiled, cook them fifteen to twenty minutes. An egg boiled seven or eight minutes is not only hard but tough. Longer boiling makes the albumin mellow. Always prepare eggs simply without using grease.

Eggs may be given in combination with either fruits or vegetables. Milk is not to be taken in the egg meal, for if such combinations are made the child gets more protein than necessary. Eggs are easy to digest and the chief objection to their free use in feeding children is that the protein intake will be too great, which causes disease.

Nuts should not be given until the children are old enough to masticate them thoroughly. The best combination is the same as for eggs. Children under six years of age should not have much more than one-half of an ounce of nut meats at a meal. The pecans are the best. Children rarely chew nuts well enough, so they should seldom be used. They may be ground very fine and made into nut butter, which may be substituted for ordinary butter.

Give no butter until the child has completed his second year. The whole milk contains all the fat necessary. Butter should always be used in moderation, for although it digests easily, it is a very concentrated food.

Again the question will be asked: "How much shall I feed my child?" I do not know, but I do know that most children get at least three times as much food as is good for them. People can establish a toleration to a certain poison, and seemingly take it with impunity for a while. Some arsenic eaters and morphine addicts take enough of their respective drugs daily to kill a dozen normal men. However, the drugs, if not stopped, always ruin the user in the end. It is the same way with food. Children seem to establish a toleration for an excess for a shorter or longer period of time, but the overeating always produces discomfort and disease in the end, and if it is continued it will cause premature death.

About one-third or one-fourth of what children eat is needed to nourish them. The rest makes trouble. Read the chapters in this book on overeating and on normal food intake. They give valuable pointers. Parents know their children best, and the mother can, or should be able to tell when there are signs of impending danger. If there is a decided change in the child's disposition it generally denotes illness. Some children become very sweet when they are about to be ill, but most of them are so cranky that they make life miserable for the family. A foul, feverish breath nearly always comes before the attack. A common danger signal is a white line around the mouth. Another one is a white, pinched appearance of the nose. A flushed face is quite common. The tongue never looks normal. Except the abnormal tongue, these symptoms are not all present before every attack, but one or more of them generally are. No matter what the signs of trouble may be, stop all feeding immediately. If this is done, the disease generally fails to develop, but if feeding is continued there is sure to be illness. These symptoms indicate that the digestion is seriously disturbed. It is folly to feed when there is an acute attack of indigestion. Besides, it is very cruel, for it causes much suffering.

Such symptoms in children are caused by improper eating, and overeating is generally the chief fault. The remedy is very simple: Feed less.

A coated tongue indicates too much food. A clean tongue shows that the digestive organs are working well. If the tongue is not smooth and a pretty pink in color, it means that the child has had too much food and the meals must be reduced in quantity until the tongue does become normal, which may take a few months in chronic cases. Peculiar little protruding spots when red and prominent on the tip and edges of the tongue indicate irritation of the alimentary tract and call for reduction of food intake.

The parents can soon learn how much to feed the children if they will be guided by these hints. Poor health in the children indicates parental failure, and this is one place where they can not afford to fail. Parents must be honest with themselves and not put the blame where the doctors put it--on bacteria, draughts, the weather, etc. Sometimes the climate is very trying on the babies, but it never kills those who have intelligent care.

If it is found that the child next door, of the same age, eats three or four times as much as your child, do not become alarmed about your little one, but give the neighbor's child a little silent sympathy because its parents are ignorant enough to punish the little one so cruelly.

For those who desire more definite hints regarding feeding of children, an outline has been prepared for several days. This is very simple feeding, but it is the kind of feeding that will make a rose bloom in each cheek. The child will be happy and contented and bring joy to the hearts of the parents.

Breakfast: Whole wheat toast, butter and a glass of milk.

Lunch: A baked apple and a dish of cottage cheese.

Supper: Steamed or boiled brown rice and milk.

Breakfast: Puffed wheat and milk.

Lunch: Oranges and milk.

Supper: An egg, parsnips and onions, both stewed.

Breakfast: Oatmeal or whole wheat porridge and milk.

Lunch: Berries and milk.

Supper: Baked potato, spinach and a plate of lettuce.

Breakfast: Shredded wheat biscuit and milk.

Lunch: Stewed prunes and milk or cottage cheese.

Supper: Whole wheat toast and milk.

These are merely hints. Where one juicy fruit is suggested, another may be substituted. In place of the succulent vegetables named, others may be used. Any of the starches may be selected in place of the ones given. However, no mistake will be made in using the whole wheat products as the starch mainstay.

Desserts should not be fed to children often. Rich cakes and all kinds of pies should be omitted from the bill of fare. It is true that some children can take care of them, but what is the use of taking chances? A plain custard, lightly flavored, may be given with toast. If ice cream is above suspicion a moderate dish of this with some form of starch may be given, but milk is not to be taken in the same meal with either ice cream or custard.

At the end of the third year it is time enough to begin to feed the salad vegetables, though they may be given earlier to children who masticate well. The dressing should be very plain, nothing more than a little salt and olive oil, or some clabbered cream. No dressing is necessary. The salad vegetables may be eaten with the meal containing eggs and the stewed succulent vegetables.

At the age of about seven or eight the child may be put on the same diet as the parents, provided they live simply. Otherwise, continue in the old way a little longer. For the best results in raising children, simplicity is absolutely necessary.

Children who are early put on a stimulating diet develop mental and sexual precocity, both of which are detrimental to physical welfare. The first desideratum is to give the children healthy bodies, and then there will be no trouble in giving them what knowledge they need.

In overfed boys the sex urge is so strong that they acquire secret habits, and sometimes commit overt acts. Too much protein is especially to blame. These facts are not understood by many and the result is that the parents fail in their duty to their children.

It is best not to bring young children to the table, if there is anything on it that they should not have, for it nearly always results in improper feeding. The children are curious and they beg for a little of this and a little of that. Unthinkingly the parents give them little tastes and bites and before the meal is over they have had from six to twelve different kinds of food, some of them not fit for adult consumption. If the child understands that it is not to ask for these things and abides by this rule, it is all right, but such children are rare. A child that fretfully begs for this and that at the table upsets itself and the parents.

Make no sudden changes in the manner of feeding, unless the feeding is decidedly wrong.

Active children get all the exercise they need. They should spend a large part of the day in the open, and this is even more important for the delicate ones. The bedroom should be well ventilated, but the children must be kept cozy and warm or they do not sleep well.

After the child is old enough not to soil itself, one or two baths a week are sufficient. There is no virtue in soaking. Swimming is different, for here the child is active in the water and it does not weaken him so. Swimming should be a part of every child's education.

Bed time should be early. The children should be tucked in and the light turned off by 8 o'clock, and 7 o'clock is better for children under five. If they want to get up early in the morning, let them, but put them to bed early at night.

Infants should not be exposed long to the direct rays of the summer sun, for it is liable to cause illness. It upsets the stomach and then there is a feverish spell. If nothing is fed that will generally be all, but it is unnecessary to make babies ill in this way. They should not be chilled either.

Husband and wife do not agree at all times, but they make a mistake when they disagree in the presence of their children. Young people are quick to take advantage of such a state of affairs and they begin to play the parents against each other. When a point comes up where there is a difference of opinion, the decision of the parent who speaks first should stand, at least for the time being. Then when they are by themselves, man and wife can discuss the matter if it is not satisfactory, and even quarrel about it, if that gives them pleasure. Parents who do not control themselves can not long retain the full respect of their children. Lost respect is not very far distant from lost love.

People often object to a change in methods, for, they say, the new plan will cause too much trouble. The plan here outlined causes less trouble than the conventional method of caring for children. It is simpler and gives better results. If it were followed out the mortality of children under ten years of age in this country would be reduced from over 400,000 annually to less than

25,000. In spite of everything, a number of young people will get into fatal pranks.

There are difficulties in the way of raising children properly, but a healthy child is such a great reward that the efforts are paid for a hundred times over. Nothing wears the parents out more quickly than a child who is always fretting and crying, always on the brink of disease or in its grasp. In raising children the best way is the easiest way.

THE CHILD'S MENTAL TRAINING.

A healthy body is the child's first requirement. However, if the mental training is poor, giving wrong views of life, a good physique is of but little service.

It is quite generally agreed among observers that the first seven years of life leave the mental impressions which guide the whole life, and that after the age of fourteen the mental trend rarely changes. There are a few individuals with strength enough to make themselves over mentally after reaching adult life, but these are so few that they are almost negligible, and even they are largely influenced by their youth and infancy. It is as easy to form good mental habits as bad ones. It is within the power of all parents to give their children healthy bodies and healthy minds, and this is a duty, which should prove a pleasure. The reason such heritage is so rare is that it requires considerable self-control and most parents live chaotic lives.

Upon the mentality depends the success in life. "It is the mind that makes the body rich." No matter how great an individual's success may seem in the eyes of the public, if the person lacks the proper perspective, the proper vision and the right understanding, his success is an empty thing. Wealth and success are considered synonymous, but I have found more misery in the homes of the rich than among the poor. Physical wants can be supplied and the suffering is over, but mental wants can only be satisfied through understanding, which should be cultivated in childhood.

"All our problems go back to the child--corrupt politics, dishonesty and greed in commerce, war, anarchism, drunkenness, incompetence and criminality."--Moxom.

Given a healthy body and a good mind, every individual is able to become a useful member of society, and that is all that can be expected of the average individual. All can not be eminent, and it is not necessary.

Upon the child's mental impressions and the habits formed in infancy and youth depend the mental workings and the habits of later life. Therefore it is necessary to nurture the little people in the right kind of atmosphere. If the child is trained properly from infancy there will be no serious bad habits to overcome during later years, and, as all know, habits are the hardest of all bonds to break. To overcome the coffee and alcohol habits is hard, but to overcome bad mental habits is even more difficult.

First of all, let the infant alone most of the time. Some mothers are so full of love and nonsense that they take their babies up to cuddle and love them at short intervals, and then there are the admiring relatives who like to flatter the parents by telling them that the baby is the finest one they have seen; it is an exceptional baby. So the relatives have to bother the infant and kiss it. This should not be. The child should be kept in a quiet room and should not be disturbed. There are no exceptional babies. They are all much alike, except that some are a little healthier than others. If they are let alone, they have the best opportunity to develop into exceptional men and women.

Paying too much attention to babies makes them cross and irritable. They soon learn to like and then to demand attention. If they do not get it at once they become ill-tempered and cry until attention is given. Thus the foundation of bad temper is laid in the very cradle. They gain their ends in infancy by crying. Later on they develop the whining habit. When they grow older they fret and worry. Such dispositions are the faults of the parents.

It does not take long for children to learn how to get their way, and if they can do it by being disagreeable, you may be sure that they will develop the worst side of their nature. Let the child understand that being disagreeable buys nothing, and there will soon be an end of it. Children who are well and well cared for are happy. They cause their elders almost no trouble. To lavish an excessive amount of care on a baby may be agreeable to the mother at first, but it is different when it comes to caring for an ill-tempered, spoiled child of eight or nine years.

Many crimes are committed in the name of love. Many babies are killed by love. Unless love is tempered by understanding it is as lethal as poison. Many parents think they are showing love when they indulge their children, but instead they are putting them onto the road that leads to physical and mental decay. True love is helpful, kind and patient. The spurious kind is noisy, demonstrative and impatient.

Do what is necessary for children, but do not allow them to cause unnecessary work. What they can do for themselves they should do. They can be taught to be helpful very early. They should be taught to be neat and tidy. They should learn to dress themselves and how to keep their rooms and personal effects in good order early in life, no matter how many servants there may be. These little things are reflected in their later lives. They help to form the individual's character. It is what we do that largely make us what we are, and every little act and every thought has a little influence in shaping our lives. An orderly body helps to make an orderly mind and vice versa.

Many of the rich children are unfortunate indeed. Some times poor parents have so many children that each one gets scant attention, but the children of many of the rich get no parental attention. The parents are too busy accumulating or preserving a fortune and climbing a social ladder to bother with their children. Their raising is delegated to servants. At times the little ones are put on display for a few minutes and then the parents are as proud of them as they are of the expensive paintings that adorn the walls or the blooded dogs and horses in kennels and stables. No amount of paid service can compensate for the lack of parental love.

The ideal today, especially for female children, seems to be to make ornaments of them, to train them to be useless. Girls, as well as boys, should be taught to be useful. They should be taught that those who do not labor are parasites. If some do not work, others have to work too hard. The story is told of Mark Twain that he dined with an English nobleman who boasted that he was an earl and did not labor. "In our country," said Mark Twain, "we do not call people of your class earls; we call them hoboes."

It does not matter how wealthy parents are, they should teach their children how to earn a living, and they should instill into them the ideal of service, for a life of idleness is a failure. The shirkers and wasters are not happy. The greatest contentment in life comes from the performance of good work. Ecstatic love and riotous pleasure can not last. Work with love and pleasure is good. But love and pleasure without work are corroding.

Children who are waited upon much become selfish. They soon become grafters, expecting and taking everything and giving nothing. This is immoral, for life is a matter of compensation, and consists in giving as well as in taking. Children should be taught consideration for others, and should not be allowed to order the servants around; not that it harms the servants, but it has a bad effect on the children.

Because the child's period of development is so long, it is important to have a proper adjustment in the home between parents and the children. Lack of adjustment wears out the parents, especially the mother, and gives false impressions to the young people. To prevent friction and get good results, children should be taught obedience. Obedience is one of the stepping stones to ability to command.

In those homes where the words of the parents are law there is but little friction. Obedience should be taught from the very start. As soon as the child realizes that the parents mean what they say and that it is useless to fret and complain about a command, that is the end of the matter. How different it is with disobedient children! The parents have to tell them what to do several times and then the bidding often remains undone.

Begin to teach obedience and promptness as soon as the children understand, for it is more difficult later. The older the children the harder it is. Children know so little and are so conceited that they do not realize that because of lack of experience, observation and reflection they can not safely guide themselves at all times. When they are allowed to act so that they are a nuisance to others and harmful to themselves, they do not give up this license with good grace. There are times to be firm and then firmness should be used. It is necessary for the parents to cooperate.

Various parents have different ways of correcting their children, and it is not difficult to make them realize that obedience is a part of the plan of early life. To illustrate: If the children are called for a meal, they should come promptly.

If there is a tendency to lag, tell them that if they do not come when called they will get nothing to eat until next mealtime, and act accordingly. This is no cruelty, for no one is harmed by missing a meal. It generally proves very effective.

At the table, serve the children what your experience has told you they can take with benefit, without saying anything about it. If they ask for anything else, give it if you think proper. If not, say no. If they start to beg and whine, tell them that such conduct will result in their being sent away from the table, and if they still continue, do as you have said, and let there be no weakening. This may cause a few very disagreeable experiences at first, but it is much better to have a few of them and be through, than to continue year after year to have such trouble. Some children can eat everything with apparent impunity and their parents usually pay no attention to what they eat. But there are others who become ill if they are improperly fed. Children who are often feverish and take all the diseases peculiar to the young, are maltreated. They are not properly fed. Those who are prone to convulsions must be fed with great care, or there is danger of their becoming epileptics. Firmness in such cases generally means the difference between health and disease or even death.

By all means be firm in such matters. Indulging the children to excess is invariably harmful. When your children become ill and die, you can truly say, "Behold my handiwork."

In the same way teach the children to do promptly whatever they are told to do. If they are told to go to bed, it should be done without delay or protest. All the little duties that fall to their lot should likewise be accomplished promptly. However, the parents should be reasonable and they should avoid bombarding their children with commands to do or not to do a thousand and one things that do not matter at all. Let the children alone except when it is really necessary to direct them.

Unfortunately, most of the parents are blind to their own faults, but see very clearly those of others. The mistakes they make in their own families open their eyes to those of others, and then they are often very impatient. I know one gentleman who has excellent knowledge of the proper training of the young, but as a parent he is a total failure. He is so explosive and lacking in patience and firmness, perhaps also in love, that his knowledge has not helped him. It is not what we know, but what we apply, that makes or mars.

Obedience reduces friction and trains the children into habits of efficiency. It is not only valuable in preserving the health of the parents, but in increasing the child's earning capacity when the time comes to labor in earnest.

Plato said that democracies are governed as well as they deserve to be. Likewise, parents get as much obedience, respect, affection and love as they deserve, and the three latter are largely dependent upon the former. It would be difficult to overemphasize the importance of obedience.

In nature we find that the animals teach their young how to live independently as soon as they have the strength to care for themselves. This is what parents should teach their children. This may cause the mother pain, for many mothers like to keep their children helpless, dependent and away from contact with the world as long as possible. Wise mothers do not handicap their children thus. The best parents are those who teach their children early how to make their own way.

Doubtless the greatest happiness is to be found in a congenial family, where the parents understand and love each other and their children. Those parents who are so busy that they lack the time to become acquainted with their infants and keep up this intimacy, are losing a part of life that neither money nor social position can give them. Many wait until too late to get on intimate terms with their children. When young, the children are naturally loving and then the beautiful ties which neither time nor misfortune can sunder are formed. When the children are grown it is too late to establish such a relation. Then they look at their parents with as critical eyes as they use toward other people, and though they may become very good friends, the tender love is lacking. Love between man and woman is unstable, but the beautiful love that springs from companionship of children and parents lasts until the end.

While some mothers neglect their children, many become too absorbed in them. The children become all of the mother's life. As the young people become older, their horizon naturally widens. During infancy the parents can fill the child's whole life, but soon other interests crave attention. There is always a tragedy in store for the mother who refuses to see that her children, as they grow older, will demand the human experience necessary for individual growth and development. If the mother has no other interest than her children she will one day be left with a heart as empty as the home from which the children are gone. There are so many interesting things in this world, and every mother should have her hobby. She should have at least one hour each day sacred to herself, in which she can relax and cultivate the mind. This will help to fill the coming years, which too often prove barren. Loving parents get all the reward they should expect from the beautiful intimacy that exists between them and their growing children. So-called ungrateful children have incompetent parents. Parents have no right to demand gratitude. They do no more for their children than was done for themselves in the morning of their lives. The right kind of parents never want for rewards. They are repaid every day so long as they live. Children grow under the care of their parents, but the parents also grow and expand in understanding, sympathy and love through association with their children.

Today society does not treat the mothers with the proper consideration. The mothers deserve well, for they have to give many of their best years to the children. These are the productive years, and generally unfit the women to go into economic competition with the rest of the world afterwards. Society owes it to the mothers of the race to see that they are not made to suffer for fulfilling their destiny. Motherhood today is as dangerous as the soldier's life, though it ought not to be, and it is more difficult to raise children than to conduct a successful business. However, the financial rewards for motherhood are generally nil. The least society can do is to see that these women do not want for the necessities of life.

Most children are interrogation points. This is well, for they learn through curiosity. The questions should be answered honestly, or not at all. It is common to give untrue answers. This is poor policy, for the answers are a part of the child's education and untruths make the young people ignorant and superstitious. It takes considerable patience to raise a child and he who is unwilling to exercise a little patience has no right to become a parent.

Whether to use corporeal punishment or not is a question that the parents must decide for themselves. Many parents are in the habit of nagging their children. It is, "Don't do this," and "Don't do that," until the little ones feel as exasperated as the Americans in Berlin, where everything that one has an impulse to do is "Verboten." The children have not yet acquired caution, nor are they able to think of more than one or two things at a time. Consequently they forget what they are not to do, and then parental wrath descends upon them. Parents can well afford to be deaf and blind to many things that happen. Those mothers who are ever shouting prohibitions soon cultivate a fretful, irritable tone that is bad for all concerned, and which does not breed respect and obedience. Make it a rule not to interfere with the children except when it is necessary, and tell them to do but one thing at a time.

If too many commands and prohibitions are issued, the children are prone to forget them all. If they are talked to less, what is said is more deeply impressed on their minds, and the chances are that they will remember. Boisterousness is not badness, but indicates a state of well-being, which results in bodily activity, including the use of the vocal cords. It is common to all young animals, and the human animal is the only one that is severely punished for manifesting happiness.

If the parents decide that corporeal punishment is necessary, they should be sure that it has been deserved, for a child resents being punished unjustly, and undeserved punishment is always harmful. Many parents become so angry that they inflict physical punishment to relieve their own feelings, and this is very wrong. If a parent calmly decides that his child needs punishment, perhaps this is the case. The punishment should be given calmly. Nothing can be more cowardly and disgusting than the brutal assault of an angry parent upon a defenseless child, and such parents always regret their actions if they have any conscience, but they are generally of such poor moral fibre and so full of false pride that they fail to apologize to the children for the injustice done. These parents inflict suffering upon their children, but they punish themselves most of all, for they kill filial regard and love. Children have a very keen sense of fair play.

If it is decided to administer corporeal punishment, it should have enough sting to it so that it will be remembered. Parents who temper their justice with patience and love are not compelled to resort to corporeal punishment often.

Children should never be hit on the head. Pulling or boxing the ears should not be recognized as civilized warfare. Blows on the head may partly destroy the hearings and affect the brain.

Another thing that may not come under the head of punishment in the strictest sense, is lifting children by one of the arms. Women are prone to do this. Often it partly dislocates the elbow joint. The children whine and no one knows exactly what is the matter. If one arm is occupied and the child has to be lifted from curb to street or over a puddle, stoop and pass the unoccupied arm about the child's body and no harm will be done.

No one should suggest to the child that it is bad. It is better to dwell upon goodness. If a child is often told that it is bad, it will soon begin to live up to its name and reputation, just as adults often do.

Many parents are in the habit of scaring their children. If the little ones cry or disobey, they are told that the boogy-man is coming after them, or they are threatened with being put out into the dark, or perhaps some animal or bad person is coming to get them. Fear is injurious to everybody, being ruinous to both the body and the mind, and it is especially bad for growing children. The fear instilled in them during childhood remains with some people to the end of life. It is not uncommon to find people who dare not go out alone after dark because they were scared in childhood. Children like exciting stories that would naturally inspire fear, but it is not difficult for the reader or story teller to inform the little ones that there are no big black bears or bold robbers in the neighborhood, and that now there is nothing to fear in the darkness.

Many teach the children to be ashamed of their bodies. Every part of the body has its use and whatever is useful is good. Those who do not abuse their bodies have nothing of which to be ashamed.

The education of children in the past has been along wrong lines. It has been the aim to cram them full of isolated facts, many of them untrue. We are slowly outgrowing this tendency, but too much remains. Thanks largely to Froebel and Doctor Montessori, our methods are growing more natural. The adult learns by doing and so does the child. Doctor Montessori teaches the children to use all their senses. She gives them fabrics of various textures and objects of different shapes and colors. Thus they learn colors, forms, smoothness, roughness, etc. She teaches them how to dress and undress and how to take their baths. She lets them go about the schoolroom instead of compelling them to sit still at their desks in cramped positions. In this way they get knowledge that they never forget. They learn to read and write and figure in playful ways through the proper direction of their curiosity. Little tots of four, or even younger, are often able to read, and there has been no forcing. All has come about through utilizing the child's curiosity.

If children are delicate, they should not be put into a schoolroom with thirty or forty other children. Keep such children outdoors when the weather permits and allow them to become strong. The education will take care of itself later. There is nothing to be gained by overtaxing a delicate child in the schoolroom, which too often is poorly ventilated, and having a funeral a little later.

Children should be taught the few simple fundamental rules of nutrition until they are second nature. A thorough knowledge of the fact that it is very injurious to eat when there is bodily or mental discomfort is worth ten thousand times as much to a child as the ability to extract cube root or glibly recite, "Arma virumque cano Trojae," etc. The realization that underchewing and overeating will cause mental and physical degeneration is much more valuable than the ability to demonstrate that a straight line is the shortest distance between two points. This knowledge can be given so unobtrusively that the child does not realize that it is learning, for there are many opportunities.

When a child gets sick and is old enough to understand, instead of sympathizing with it explain how the illness came about, and please remember that in explaining you can leave the germs out of the question, for diseases of childhood are almost entirely due to improper feeding. The value of education like that is beyond any price, for it is a form of health insurance. Reforming the race, means that we must begin with the children.

In parts of Europe cultured people have a working knowledge of two or three languages. This is certainly convenient. Those who wish their children to know one or two tongues beside English should remember that in infancy two tongues are learned as readily as one, if they are spoken. Those who can use three languages when they are four years old are not infant prodigies. They have had the opportunity to learn, and languages are simply absorbed.

The language teaching in the public schools is a joke. After taking several years of French or German the school children can not speak about the common things of life in those tongues, though they may know more about the grammar than the natives. In other words, they know the science of the language, but not the language itself.

A time comes when the child wants to know about the origin of life. If the parents have been companions, they can impart this knowledge better than anyone else. If they are unable to explain, the family doctor should be able to impart the knowledge with delicacy. I do not believe that such knowledge should be imparted to mixed classes in the public schools, as advocated by some. If the parents do their duty, there will be no need of public education in sex hygiene.

The doctor should be an educator, so he merits consideration here. Nearly all families have their medical advisers, and these professional people have it in their power to bring more sunshine into the homes than their fees will pay for. On the other hand, they can, and too often do, give both advice and remedies that are harmful They should sow seeds of truth. If the infant is properly cared for, it is never ill. Inasmuch as there are but few families with sufficient knowledge to keep their babies healthy at all times, there are many calls for the doctor. Parents are generally unduly alarmed about their infants. Nearly always the trouble is primarily in the alimentary tract, due to improper feeding, and the doctor with his wide experience can relieve the parental anxiety, and at the same time tell them where they have made their mistakes and how they have brought suffering upon their little ones.

Of course, there should be no dosing with medicine and no injections of foreign matter into the blood stream. Rest, quiet, cleanliness and warmth are what the children need to restore them to health. The right kind of physician when acting as adviser to intelligent parents who wish to do the best by their children will see to it that there is little or no disease.

If the parents do not know what to do, the most economical procedure is to consult a physician who has understanding of and confidence in nature. Pay no attention to the women of many words who give advice "because they have had many children and have buried them all."

It is not as difficult to raise healthy children as sickly ones. It is so simple that it takes many pages to explain it.

CHAPTER XXVIII.

DURATION OF LIFE.

Old age today brings to mind a picture of decrepitude and decay. This is because there is practically no natural old age. Those who live so that they are unhealthy during the early years of life will not be well if they reach advanced years. Old people can be well in body and sound in mind. In order to attain this desirable end, it is necessary to live properly during the first part of life. It is true that people may dissipate and reform and then live long in comfort, but usually those who spend too lavishly destroy their capital and go into physical or mental bankruptcy.

There are many who during their prime say that they do not wish to grow old. Their desire for a short life can easily be satisfied. All that is necessary is to live in the conventional manner and the chance of dying before reaching the age of fifty or sixty is good. A few live to be seventy or more in spite of dissipation, but these are the exceptions. They were endowed with excellent constitutions to begin with, constitutions that were made to last over one hundred years. Where we find one who has lived long in spite of intemperance, thousands have died from it.

Most people desire to remain on earth long and they can have their wish. They can advance in years healthy in body and with growing serenity of mind. Physical and mental well-being are necessary to attain one's life's expectancy. Old age should not be considered as apart from the rest of life. It is but one of the natural phases. Those who do not live to be old have failed to live completely.

Those who express their desire to die young generally change their mind when they face death. Man clings to life.

Old age is a desirable condition. The physical tempests have been subdued, if the life has been well spent. On the other hand, the faults and foibles of the self-indulgent are accentuated and in such cases old age is a misfortune.

No one knows what man's natural length of life is. Anatomists and physiologists compare the human body with the bodies of various animals. In this they are justified, for we all develop according to the same laws. Most of the animals, when allowed to live as nature intended them to live, reach an age of from five to six times the length of the period of their growth. Human beings, with their ability to control their environment, should be able to do even better than that. Man reaches physical maturity between twenty and twenty-five years of age. This would make his natural age one hundred and twenty-five to one hundred and fifty years. There are cases on record that have lived longer and it may be that if man would cease going in the way of self-destruction and spend more thought and time on the welfare of the race, life would be prolonged beyond even one hundred and fifty years. R. T. Trall, M. D., thought that man should live to be two hundred years old.

"What man has done man can do." If long life is worth while, doubtless a time will come when long life will be enjoyed. The worry, fretting and foolish haste of today will doubtless be partly done away with some time. Then men and women will have time to live, instead of merely existing, as most people do today. Men have lived long and found life good. Long life for its own sake is perhaps not to be desired, but the benefit that can be bestowed upon the race by those advanced in years is desirable. Occasionally a brilliant individual appears on the scene, doing superior work in life's morning, but most of the work that has been found worthy of the consideration of the ages has been done by men of mature years.

Galen, the famous physician, is said to have lived to a great age. It is hard to tell exactly how old he was, but he was probably well past the century mark at his death. His long life gave him time to do work that is appreciated after the lapse of eighteen centuries. For many hundred years after his death he dominated the practice of medicine and he is today spoken of as often as any living medical man.

Thomas Parr, an Englishman, died at the age of one hundred and fifty-two. He was hale and hearty to the very end. Unfortunately, his reputation traveled far. He was brought to the English court, where he was wined and dined, and as a consequence he died. Before this he had always led the simple life. An autopsy was performed and the physicians found his organs in excellent condition. The only reason they could give for his death was his departure from the simple life which he had led in his home.

Henry Jenkins, also an Englishman, lived to the age of one hundred and sixty-nine years. He lived very frugally and was always on friendly terms with nature. His favorite drink was water, though he partook in moderation of "hop bitters." He was moderate in all things, and it is said that he was never really ill until near the end of life. He was not shriveled and shrunken, but a wholesome looking man. King Charles II. sent a carriage to bring Mr. Jenkins to London, when he was one hundred and sixty years old. The old gentleman declined to ride and walked the two hundred miles to the metropolis. The king questioned him regarding his life and desired to know the reason for his longevity. Mr. Jenkins replied that he had always been sober and temperate and that this was the reason for his many years. The Merry Monarch was neither sober nor temperate, and you may be sure that this reply did not please him. Mr. Jenkins was wiser than Mr. Parr had been, refusing to dissipate, even though he was old. Consequently he returned to his home to enjoy life nine years longer.

These two cases are authentic.

All are familiar with the records given in the Bible. Whether they are figurative or not it is hard to tell. However, so many cases of longevity are recorded that they in all probability have a basis in fact. The Hebrews of old must have been a long-lived people. One hundred and twenty years was not an extreme age. In Genesis is the record of many over five hundred years old, and a few over nine hundred years of age. At the time of the apostles the life span of the Hebrews had grown shorter and hence the dictum of three score years and ten. Between the time of Moses and that of the apostles the Hebrews had advanced--or shall we say degenerated?--from a semi-barbarous people to one that had the graces and also the vices of a higher civilization. The Hebrews of old were husbandmen, who lived simply and got their vigor from the soil.

The cause of so much unnecessary suffering and of the premature deaths has been discussed elsewhere in this book. In short, it is wrong living and wrong thinking. Impure air and bad food kill no more surely than does worry.

The bodies of children are composed largely of water. The structures are flexible and elastic. The bones are made up mostly of cartilaginous structure. As the children grow older more solids are deposited in the body and the proportion of solid matter to water grows greater. Lime is deposited in the bones. When they are limy throughout they are said to be ossified. After this process is complete no more growth can take place. Bone formation continues until about the age of twenty-five. At this age the body is efficient. The fluids circulate without obstruction. Could this condition be maintained, there would be no decay.

During the early years of life the food intake in proportion to the weight of the body is great. The child is active and uses much fuel to produce power and to repair the waste. Considerable food is required for body building. At this time a broken bone mends quickly and cuts heal in a short time. With advancing years come slowness and sluggishness of the various vital activities. The slowing up can be retarded almost indefinitely by proper care of the body.

If the circulation could be maintained and the purity of the blood stream guarded, old age would be warded off. A healthy body is able to cleanse itself under favorable conditions and so long as the body is clean through and through there is no opportunity for disease to take place and there can be no aging. By aging I mean not so much the number of years one has lived as the amount of hardening and degeneration of the body that take place.

Some are as old at forty as others are at seventy.

When people have reached physical maturity they should begin to reduce their food intake. There is no need for building material then. All that is necessary is enough to repair the waste and to keep up the temperature. The individual at twenty-seven should eat a little less than when he was twenty and by the age of thirty-five he should have reduced his food still more and made his meals very simple. Children enjoy the gratification of the sense of taste, but at the age of thirty-five a man has lived enough and experienced enough so that he should know that the overgratification of appetites is an evanescent and unprofitable pleasure, always costing more than it is worth. It is best to grow into good habits while young, for it is difficult to do so after one has grown old. The man who reforms after fifty is the exception.

Children are fond of cereal foods and sugars. They can eat these foods two or three times a day and thrive. A man of thirty-five should make it a general rule to limit his starch eating to once a day. Various physiologists say that as much as sixteen ounces of dry starch (equivalent to about thirty ounces of ordinary bread) are necessary each day. This is entirely too much. Very few people can profitably eat more than four ounces of dry starch a day, and for many this is too much. Through eating as much as is popularly and professionally advocated, early decay and death result.

The arteries are normally pliable and elastic. When too much food is taken, the system is unable to cleanse itself. Debris is left at various points. One of the favorite lodging places is in the coats of the arteries. After considerable deposits have been formed the arteries lose their elasticity. They become hard and unyielding. A normal radial artery can easily be compressed with one finger. Sometimes the radial artery becomes so hard that it is difficult to compress it with three fingers. As the arteries grow harder they become more brittle and sometimes they break, often a fatal accident.

This hardness of the arteries impedes the circulation, for the tone and natural elasticity of the vessel walls is one of the aids to a normal circulation.

So long as the arteries are normal all parts of the body are bathed in a constantly changing stream of blood. The muscles, the nerves, the bones, in fact all parts of the body, remove from the blood stream those elements that are necessary for repairing or building the various tissues. They also throw into the blood stream the refuse and waste due to the constant repair and combustion going on all over the body. The blood then leaves this refuse with the skin, lungs, kidneys and bowels, which throw it out of the body.

So long as there are enough fuel and food, but not too much, and so long as all the debris is carried away, there is health. But let this process be thrown out of balance and there will be disease. The food intake is seldom too small, though the digestion is frequently so poor that not enough good food gets into the blood. Old age is largely due to overeating and eating the wrong kinds of food. This is how overeating causes premature aging, when it does not kill more quickly: When too much food is taken, too much is absorbed into the blood, provided the nutritive processes are active. Then all the food in the blood can not be used for repair and fuel. The balance must either be excreted or stored away in the body as deposits. If this storing takes place in the joints, the result may be rheumatism or gout and at times even a complete locking of the joints (anchylosis). If it is stored in the walls of the blood-vessels they become hard and unyielding. No matter where deposits take place, some of them will be found in the walls of the blood-vessels. When these vessels grow hard they decrease in caliber. The result is that the heart is compelled to work very hard, but even then enough blood is not forced through the vessels. The circulation becomes sluggish. The blood in the various parts becomes stagnant.

Then insufficient good oxygen and first-class nourishment are brought to the parts and not enough waste is carried away. Now the billions of cells of which the body is composed are constantly bathed in poisonous blood. The result is lowering of physical tone, or degeneration, of the whole body. The hands and the feet suffer most at first from the poor blood supply and become cold easily. Those who suffer constantly from cold hands and feet should know that they are aging, although they may be but twenty years old.

Such a condition as this often gives rise to varicose veins in the legs. The feet are so far away from the heart, and it is such a long upgrade return of the blood, that the circulation in the lower extremities easily becomes sluggish. The flabby, relaxed tissues and the hardened blood-vessels allow the blood to stagnate. This is why senile gangrene is so common in the feet and so often fatal.

The brain gets a copious blood supply, yet the hardening of the arteries often deprives this organ of its necessary nourishment. Then the higher faculties begin to abdicate. If the hardening is extensive senile softening of the brain may take place. This is always due to a lack of pure blood. Sometimes the arteries are brittle enough to break. Baldness is another symptom of physical decay. The hair follicles are not properly nourished, for the arteries have become so contracted and the tissues of the scalp so hardened that there is not enough blood to feed the hair roots. Baldness begins on top of the head, generally the only part affected, because it is farthest away from the blood supply. Baldness is also partly due to man's headwear. Women are rarely bald. There is a saying that there are no bald men in the poorhouse. Even if this were true, it would not be very consoling, for the bald heads on the street cleaning forces are numerous.

Overeating also causes premature aging because if results in fermentation in the alimentary tract. The acids produced cause degeneration of various tissues, having an especially bad effect on the nervous system, which reflects the evil to other parts of the body.

It is well to bear in mind how this comes about: First there is overeating; too much food improperly prepared is taken into the blood stream; this makes the blood impure; deposits, causing hardening of the tissues and reduction of the lumen of the vessels, are formed; the blood grows more impure and the circulation sluggish; the tissues are constantly bathed in impure blood, causing further degeneration. When a certain point is reached nature can tolerate no more and life flits away.

Those who wish to remain young must give some thought to the selection of their food, especially if they are hearty eaters. If only sufficient food is taken to keep the body well nourished it does not make much difference what is eaten, provided it contains sufficient of fresh foods, for when only enough food is taken to supply fuel and repairing material, the food will all be used and none is left to ferment in the digestive tract and form deposits in the body. The body will then keep itself clean, or at least the formation of deposits takes place so slowly that it is hardly perceptible. This can be compared with the process taking place in the flues of a boiler. Stoke properly and they remain clean. Choke the firebox with an excess of coal and the combustion is so incomplete that the flues are soon filled up and the grates are often burned out. Just so with the body: Feed too heavily and the digestive organs are burned by the abnormal amount of acid produced and the blood-vessels are filled with debris.

As most people lack the self-control to eat a normal amount of food, they should select foods that are compatible and that are not too concentrated. Too much meat causes degeneration of all parts of the body and hardening. Too much starch causes acidity and hardening. The fruits and the light vegetables have a tendency to overcome these degenerating processes.

Starch is surely the chief offender in aging people. It is such a concentrated food that overeating is easy, especially when it is taken in the soft forms, such as mushes, fresh bread, griddle cakes and mashed potatoes. If people would masticate their starchy foods thoroughly it would greatly reduce the danger of overeating. It is common to eat bread three times a day and in addition to take potatoes once or twice a day. Those who consume so much starch carry into the system more food than can be used and more of the mineral salts than can be excreted. The result is the formation of deposits, chiefly of lime carbonate and lime phosphate; fatty deposits are also common.

In order to live long and comfortably it would be well to reduce the starch intake to once a day. The meats also are objectionable when taken in excess. To them can be attributed the chief blame for the formation of gelatinous deposits in the body. However, they do not carry so much earthy matter into the blood stream as do the starches. It is best to partake of meat but once a day, or even more seldom. Meat should certainly not be taken more than twice a day even by those who are advanced in years. People who care enough for starch to take it three times a day, or are compelled to live chiefly upon it, grow old and homely more quickly than do those who are able to partake more plentifully of the more expensive proteins. The flesh obtained from young animals and birds is not so heavily charged with earthy matters as is that which is obtained from old animals and birds.

Fruits and nuts do not carry so much earthy matter as do the starches and meats. The sweet fruits could with profit partly take the place of the starchy foods. The sugar they contain, which has the same nutritive value as starches, needs very little preparation before entering the blood stream. Thus a large part of the energy required for starch digestion is saved. On the other hand, the use of too much refined sugar is even worse than an excessive intake of starch. Nuts are not difficult to digest if they are well masticated..

The objection to acid fruits during the latter years of life is that they thin the blood and cause chilliness. This is true if they are partaken of too liberally. It is not necessary to refrain from eating acid fruits, but they should be taken in moderation and the mild ones should be selected. Pears, mild apples and grapes are better than oranges, grapefruits and apricots. Those who have learned moderation can eat all the fruit desired, for they will not be harmed by what a normal appetite craves.

Vegetables carry considerable earthy matter, but on account of their helpfulness in keeping the blood sweet they should be eaten several times a week.

Those who think that overeating of starch is too harshly condemned are referred to the horse. When he is allowed to roam about and partake of his natural food, grass, he stays well and lives to be forty or more years old. When compelled to eat great quantities of corn and oats, which are very rich in starch, the horse becomes listless and slow at an early age. He is old at fifteen and before twenty he is generally dead. When horses suffer from stiffness in the joints a few weeks spent in pasture, where they have nothing but green grass and water, remove the stiffness and make them younger. This shows what partaking of nature's green salad does for them. Any good stock man will tell you that feeding too much grain "burns a cow out." It does exactly the same for a human being, burns him out and fills him with clinkers. Many people think that it is a hardship to be moderate in eating and drinking, but it is not. It brings such a feeling of well-being and comfort that it is unbelievable to those who have not experienced it.

Many envy the rich, thinking that they can and do live riotously. Rich men must live as simply as though they were poor or else they soon lose the mental efficiency that brought them their fortunes, for when health is gone mental power is reduced.

According to information in the Saturday Evening Post, the eating habits of many of our most influential business men are very simple and the amount of food partaken of small. John D. Rockefeller could hardly live more simply and plainly than he does. William Rockefeller, George F. Baker, James Stillman, Otto H. Kahn, Thomas Fortune Ryan, George W. Perkins, J. Ogden Armour, John H. Patterson, Jacob H. Schiff and Andrew Carnegie, all business giants with money enough to subsist on the most expensive delicacies, are said to live more plainly than does the average American who is complaining of the high cost of living. It is the price they have had to pay for success and it is the price that you and I will have to pay to live successfully, though our success may not take the form of financial power.

The one conspicuous exception among the financially great to the rule of simplicity was J. P. Morgan. His eating habits were somewhat gross, but on account of his rugged constitution he lived to be more than seventy-five years old. If he had given himself just a little more care he would be alive today.

They say that his strong black cigars did him no apparent harm, but those who read of his last illness understandingly cannot agree to that statement. Mr. Morgan started with enough vitality to live and work far beyond the century mark. John D. Rockefeller was not physically strong when young. He has been compelled to take good care of himself and to be moderate. Now he is past seventy and enjoying good health.

John W. Gates died a martyr to excess, partly excess of food. He lacked balance. His son followed in his footsteps and died young.

Frank A. Vanderlip, who is looming large on the financial horizon takes but two meals a day, from which he gets enough sustenance to do good work and he says that this plan makes for efficiency. Perhaps now that such men as Mr. Vanderlip live well on two meals a day, it is time to cease calling those who live thus faddists. Eating three meals a day is a habit and many can and do get along very well on two meals, and a few take only one meal daily.

E. H. Harriman also lived simply. He illustrates the evil of a poorly controlled mind. He died when but little past sixty, probably because his frail body was too weak to harbor his great ambition. He took his business wherever he went. When ill and business was forbidden by his physician, Mr. Harriman had a telephone concealed in his bedroom and as soon as the doctor was gone, he was on the wire.

Another cause of premature aging is the drinking of very hard water. The earthy matter is absorbed into the blood stream with the water, and a part of it is deposited in the various tissues. People beyond middle age should drink water containing only a small portion of salts. Those who partake of fresh fruits or fresh vegetables daily get all the salts that the system needs. Even the young should not drink water that is exceedingly hard. We can well illustrate the harm that comes from the excessively hard water by referring to the disease known as cretinism. This disease is quite prevalent in some parts of Europe. They say that the disease is hereditary, which is questionable. What is inherited is the environment and the habits of the parents. The chief cause is without doubt the superabundance of earthy matter in the drinking water. The cretins are ill-favored in face and figure. They do not reach normal mental or physical maturity. They are old long before the normal person has reached his prime. They die young, rarely living to be over thirty years old.

The bones are completely ossified early, which is the cause of their small stature and their stupidity. The bones of the skull harden so early that the brain has no room to expand.

There is no need of suffering, even in a mild degree, from the disease of cretinism. If the water is very hard it is easy to distill what is needed for drinking purposes. Such water should at least be boiled. It is much better to have a teakettle lined with earthy matters than to have such a lining in our arteries.

The excessive use of table salt is another cause of early aging. It is a good preservative and pickles meat very well. People have long used salt as a preservative and perhaps they got the salt-eating habit in this way, first using it on the foods to be preserved, and then on nearly all foods. Salts to excess, especially table salt, help to mummify or pickle those who partake of them too liberally. The addition of sodium chloride to foods is unnecessary. We get all we need of this salt in our fruits, vegetables and cereals. Salt should be used in moderation.

Alcohol, tobacco and coffee are harmful. However, it will be found that most of the old people have used one or more of these drugs for many years and this is often largely responsible for their reaching old age. Overeating causes more deaths than any other single factor. The use of tobacco, coffee or alcohol has a tendency to reduce the desire for food and thus these drugs at times prove to be conservers of individual lives, though they are undoubted racial evils. They never can or will take the place of self-control. The senses were given us to use for our protection, but most people abuse them for temporary gratification, and thus they go in the way of self-destruction.

Other things being equal, a healthy child will live longer than a weakly one. But other things are not equal, so it often happens that a weakling has as much chance to survive as a healthy person. Strong people frequently squander their inheritance by the time they are forty or fifty years old. Healthy people are very imprudent. They are well so they think they will always remain well. What a surprise it is when after thirty they discover that they cannot do with impunity what they could do before with apparently no bad results! When warned about their eating habits they boast that they can "eat tacks". Smoking and drinking are harmless, they say! But the day of reckoning always comes and the account is often so great that under the conventional treatment of today they die.

The weakling has been compelled to be careful. Habits of moderation grew upon him in youth, and his health has improved as he has advanced in years. He may never be strong, but great physical strength is not essential to health. Thus the strong often perish and the weak survive. If both classes lived with equal care the strong would outlive and outwork the weak every time.

It is necessary to give the skin some care if continued good health is desired during the latter part of life. The skin has a tendency to grow hard, which should not be allowed. It will always remain soft if it is properly cared for. When our ancestors roved forests and plains with scarcely any attire, the skin exposed to the rain and the sunshine, there was no need to give it special care. It served its purpose of protecting their bodies and was exercised through its immediate contact with the elements in all kinds of weather. Now the skin has little opportunity to exercise its protective function and the result is that it is not as active as it should be. The skin must be active to rid itself of the waste that the blood-vessels leave with it. The best exercise for this important organ is rubbing. The whole body should be rubbed every day and it would be well to do this twice a day. An occasional olive oil rub is also good. The rubbings make the body hardier. They also help to keep the circulation active and the skin smooth and soft. The blood is brought near the surface. The tendency as we grow older is for the circulation to grow less and less near the surface and in the extremities. This is slow death.

The daily rub is more important than the daily bath. If we have enough rubbing very little bathing is necessary, for an active skin cleans itself.

There are many men who have lived in the conventional way until the age of forty, fifty or sixty. They have been healthy, which means that they have been able to work most of the time, but have had their share of ills, which have incapacitated them for work or business at various times. They find after reaching a certain age that they are surely going down hill physically and that they are not as active mentally as previously. The question is, can anything be done under the circumstances? Very few of these people are in such a bad physical state that death is inevitable within the next few years. If they seek the right advice and follow it, they can generally continue to live in improved health for thirty to sixty years more.

A celebrated case in point is that of Louis Cornaro, an Italian, who died in the year 1566 at the age of one hundred and two years. In his youth he was very indiscreet and dissipated. He lived riotously until he was forty years old, and then he found himself in such poor physical condition that it was only a question of a few months until the end would come. He had everything to make life worth living, except health, so he decided to attempt to regain health and prolong his life. He quit his old life, began to live simply and instead of being a waster he became a useful citizen. We are unable to get much definite information about his habits from what he wrote but we learn that he reduced the quantity of food taken and used fewer varieties. Also, he drank sparingly of wine. He did not have any definite ideas regarding diet except that it is best to eat moderately and avoid the foods that disagree with one. In his own words: "Little by little I began to draw myself away from my disorderly life, and, little by little, to embrace the orderly one. In this manner I gave myself up to the temperate life, which has not since been wearisome to me; although, on account of the weakness of my constitution, I was compelled to be extremely careful with regard to the quality and quantity of my food and drink. However, those persons who are blessed with strong constitutions may make use of many other kinds and qualities of food and drink, and partake of them, in greater quantities, than I do; so that, even though the life they follow be the temperate one, it need not be as strict as mine, but much freer."

These sentences were written fifty or sixty years after he changed his mode of life, and show how well Mr. Cornaro realized the important fact that all people need not be treated alike. They also show that after making the change, Mr. Cornaro did not find it difficult to live simply enough to enjoy health. In nearly every instance it is temporarily disagreeable to forsake the path that is leading to death and take the one that leads to life, but after one gets used to the new way, it appears more beautiful and is more pleasant than the old.

If Cornaro had died at forty, as nearly every person situated as he was would have done, his life would have been a total loss. A few of those who were his boon companions and dissipated with him would have thought of him for a few years and regretted his early passing, for "he was a jolly good fellow." He lived a useful life, for over sixty years thereafter, and has left us in his debt for his beautiful exhortations to be temperate.

Many of the physical wrecks we meet, who will probably live from a few months to a few years more, if they continue in the old way, are in the same boat as Mr. Cornaro was at forty. They have had enough experience to begin to do good work, to be of some benefit to humanity. Instead of living and giving the world their best, they die. The world has had to educate these people, and it is expensive. Instead of living on and doing their work, they leave us when they ought to begin to repay us for what we have done for them. They are quitters.

Suppose Andrew Carnegie had died at the time he sold out his steel business. To most people he would have left an unsavory memory, for though we should have considered him successful from the business standpoint, many of us would say that the means were not justified by the end. However, Mr. Carnegie has spent many years since in furthering the cause of the spread of knowledge and in working for universal peace. Perhaps when Carnegie, the man of business, is well nigh forgotten, Carnegie, the educator, will be held in tender and thankful memory. He is now influencing the times for good and this influence will go down the ages.

A man has no right to say that he is weary of life and that he wants to die. The race has a claim on him. We learn through our mistakes. The race in general has to pay and suffer for every individual's education. When a man has acquired a measure of wisdom through experience, we have a right to claim it as our own.

Many men are wise in their own lines, but they have been so busy attending to the affairs that brought them success that they have omitted to learn how to have health. These people owe it to themselves and to humanity to take enough time to learn how to live so that they can work in health. The better the health the finer their product. Health and efficiency go hand in hand.

What is a man to do when he has reached middle age and finds himself degenerating? A man ought to know how to live at forty, but if he does not he should immediately learn. It may be true that "a man is a fool or a physician at forty," yet there is time and if a man lacks wisdom at forty he should immediately acquire some. Such an individual should get the best health adviser possible, avoiding any man who would have him take drugs. What he needs is not medicine, but to learn how to live. I am confident that the careful reader will find enough knowledge in this book to give him the key to the situation.

If the sufferer uses narcotics and stimulants, they must be stopped immediately. Even the least harmful of these, such as beer and light wine, should be avoided until good health has been won. These beverages need never be used. If they are taken rarely and in moderation they do no harm.

In every case that has come under my observation it has been necessary to simplify the food intake, that is, to reduce the quantity and the number of articles of food taken at each meal, also to simplify the cooking. The result is that the individual gets less food, but it is of better quality, for the conventional cooking spoils much of the food.

Most of these men neglect to exercise. It is necessary to be active and in the open, also to take good care of that important organ, the skin. Constipation is common, and it is a very annoying symptom, which disappears in time under proper living. The absorption of poisons from a constipated lower bowel is one of the factors that causes premature aging. When the constipation is overcome there are a feeling of physical well-being and a mental clearness which are impossible in the presence of constipation.

The treatment of such a condition is very much the same as the treatment of catarrh or any other curable disease, that is, find the errors of living and correct them.

It is really surprising how little food people need after they are fifty or sixty years old. If such people eat enough to be well nourished, but not enough to produce any bad feelings there will be no disease. People who die from disease are physical failures, for the natural end does not come in a physical upheaval. Those who live as they should will pass away without any pain. The organism simply grows weary and goes into the last sleep.

There are people who say that there needs be no physical death. Harry Gaze wrote an entertaining book on the subject some years ago and gave lectures in this country. It will not convince the average student of nature that people can live forever, for in nature there is constant change. The order of life is birth, development, reproduction, decline and death. It is not likely that man is an exception.

It is believed that in olden times men were larger and lived longer than they do today. There is not much foundation for such a belief to rest upon, except in a few cases. The last census shows that there are several thousand centenarians in the United States. In the Technical World for March, 1914, appeared an article by Byron C. Utecht, entitled, "When is Man Old?" This magazine is careful in gathering its facts. I shall quote a few paragraphs:

"Abraham Wilcox, of Fort Worth, Texas, is one hundred and twelve years old, but he takes keen enjoyment in life. He walks two miles or more every day as a constitutional and, occasionally, he even takes a small glass of beer. He looks forward with all the enthusiasm of a boy to a visit to the Panama-Pacific Exposition in 1915. Mr. Wilcox reads the newspapers every day and is interested in everything about him, from the food being prepared for his dinner to the latest feats by aeroplanes. This aged man looks forty or fifty years younger than he really is. His skin is white but not deeply lined. His vision is excellent and he walks nearly erect. Thirty years ago he gave up smoking, as his doctors warned him he was near death from old age and that the use of tobacco would only hasten the end."

"In the Ozark Mountains of Marion County, Arkansas, just across the Missouri line, lives Mrs. Elmyra Wagoner. She, too, is one hundred and twelve years old. There are a thousand wrinkles in her face and she looks her age, but in her actions she is sixty. Up until a very few years ago, when still past the hundred-year mark, Mrs. Wagoner kept a large garden and was able to work in the fields. While she has given up outdoor work, she is still active. On inclement days she sits by the fireplace in her mountain home and spins. On pleasant days she may be found walking about the yard. Recently her great-great-granddaughter was married at Protein, Missouri, six miles from the Wagoner home. This woman of one hundred and twelve years walked to the wedding, enjoyed it, and then walked back home, a distance that would tire many persons half that age. There are scores of persons at Protein who vouch for this and they tell of similar feats by Mrs. Wagoner showing remarkable physical power.

"Asked to give the causes of her longevity, the aged woman smiled and said that she hated to admit she was getting old. 'Clean, honest living, plenty of work, plenty of good food, and a desire to help others when sick or in trouble, I think gave me my long lease of life. I was always so busy caring for others and thinking of them that I never had time to worry whether I was getting old or not.'"

"Asa Goodwin, of Serrett, Alabama, is one hundred and six years old. His endurance powers are even more remarkable than those of Mrs. Wagoner or Abraham Wilcox. He walks five miles every day. He works several hours daily in his garden, eats anything he likes, and reads without glasses. His family is probably the largest in the United States. A reunion recently held in his honor was attended by eight hundred and fifty persons, three hundred and fifty being blood relatives. Goodwin has been a hunter all his life and he frequently takes down his rifle and proves that his aim is still good. He ascribes his length of life and vitality to his great interest in outdoor sport and hunting, when a young man, developing a rugged constitution that lasted him many years after he was forced to quit strenuous work because of 'old age.' He asserts that he was so busy living that he reached one hundred and six years before he realized it and wants to live fifty years more if possible. 'I feel as if I could do it, too,' he declares. 'I now can take my ease and comfort and the world looks good to me. I have always lived a temperate life, never drank, never kept late hours, and still have had as much or more fun than the average man, I think. It is only now when I have nothing to do that I get to worrying and when I find myself in that condition I take a walk or weed the garden and then feel better.'"

These people are not in what some call the higher walks of life, but they have succeeded in living, where almost all fail. They have been useful members of society, satisfied to take life as it comes, and thus they have gathered much of the sweet. They have enjoyed life, and those who enjoy give enjoyment to others. It takes an audience to make even the best of plays.

Mrs. Wagoner is not rich, but she has a philosophy that is riches enough. She knows that she receives through giving. She has lived this knowledge, which has brought blessings upon her.

These people have all led simple lives and they have worked. There is no secret about growing old gracefully. It means self-control, simple living, work for body and mind, cleanliness of body and mind, and the most important part of physical cleanliness is a clean colon. It is necessary to have a tranquil mind most of the time, for anger and worry are injurious to health.

The average span of life is lengthening. In the sixteenth century the average European did not live to be twenty years old. Now he lives to be about forty. The same increase has taken place in America. In India and China the average of life is still below twenty-four years. As civilization advances the tendency is for the average of life to lengthen, provided life does not grow so complex that knowledge is antidoted by too great artificiality.

However, it is well to note that it is not the last part of life that is being lengthened. We are allowing less and less infants to die as the years roll on. The proportion of the adult population that reaches advanced age is no greater than in the past. Our mode of life is so wrong that tuberculosis, typhoid fever, cancer, kidney diseases, pneumonia and circulatory degeneration carry off immense numbers of those whom we call middle aged, but who are really young people. These are diseases of degeneration. It is to our interest to reduce these diseases. Proper living will do it.

The life expectancy of people over fifty is even less than it was thirty years ago. Middle aged people die from diseases caused by bad habits, extended over a period of years. Therefore, these people should learn to live well if they would live longer.

The diet of the old can be about the same as that of an adult in the prime of life, except that less should be eaten. Those who live correctly have no digestive disturbances. It will be noted by those who are normal that there is not a desire for as much food as earlier in life, and this should be a guide. Old people get all the nourishment they need in two moderate meals a day. If the three-meal-a-day plan is preferred, it is all right, but then less should be taken at each meal.

White flour products are easier to digest than the whole wheat products, but normal people can digest the latter very well and it is a better food than white flour. I know one gentleman in his eighth decade of life who has grown stronger and younger by abandoning the conventional eating habits and living mostly on moderate meals of milk and whole wheat biscuits. As Cornaro said, some need more than others, but all should be moderate.

One meal a day of milk and biscuits is all right. These biscuits should be well baked and well masticated. The milk should be taken slowly.

Another meal can be meat or eggs or fish with some of the cooked and raw succulent vegetables.

If a third meal is taken, it may consist of clabbered milk or buttermilk; or of one of the sweet fruits, and the sweet fruits may be used any time in place of bread or biscuits. Cottage cheese is a good food at any time, and may be taken with fruits, either acid or sweet.

As often as desired, in summer, take fruit. Because the very acid, juicy fruits have a tendency to cause chilliness and to thin the blood, it is well to take them in moderation during advanced years, but that does not mean that those who like them should avoid them. In winter time the sweet fruit is best. Mild apples and bananas may be used as often as there is a desire for them. Oranges should be taken more rarely, as well as grapefruit, pineapples and other fruits that are heavily charged with acid.

As a general rule, the starchy foods should be eaten but once a day, but those who are very moderate may take them twice a day without bad results. Vegetarians have eggs and milk to take the place of flesh foods. They also have lentils, peas, beans and the protein in the whole wheat and other cereals. Lentils, peas and beans must be taken in moderation, for they are rich in nutriment and if too much is eaten they soon cause disease. Nuts, if well masticated, are also all right.

The general basis of feeding should be starch once a day and protein once a day in moderation. All kinds of starch and all kinds of protein may be used. Fruits more moderately than during the earlier years of life is best. All the succulent vegetables that are desired may be partaken of. By cooking the foods simply, as recommended in this book, they are rendered easier to digest than under the conventional manner of cooking. Simple cooking will help to preserve health and prolong life.

Work is one of the greatest blessings of life. Those who would live long and be useful must exercise both body and mind. Like all other blessings, if it is carried to excess it is injurious. It is unfortunate that some people must work too hard because there is a class of people who do nothing useful, being content to be wasters.

Work has been looked upon as a curse. This is a mistake. Those who live in the hope and expectation that they may some day cease working in order to enjoy life, will find when they reach the goal that life without work is not worth while. Those who can afford it can with benefit lessen the amount of productive work they do and evolve more into cultural lines, but it is dangerous to cease working. The human being is so constituted that without activity of body and mind there is degeneration. What is sadder than to see a capable individual who has won a competence and then has retired to enjoy it! He does not enjoy it. Either he has to get into some line of work, physical or mental, or he soon dies. We must have a lively interest in something or there is stagnation.

There are many beautiful things in life, and we should cultivate them while we are young enough to be able to learn to enjoy them. The loftiest spirits of the ages have left their inspirations and their aspirations with us in poetry, prose, music, painting, statuary and in other forms. We should try to cultivate understanding of these subjects, not necessarily all of them, but of one or more, for with understanding come the elevation and broadening of mind that are always present when there is sympathy, and sympathy is closely related to understanding. Culture along one or more lines broadens the mind and makes a person more worth while not only to himself, but to others. We can not estimate the value of the beauty in life in dollars and cents, but he is poor indeed who is rich in worldly goods alone.

It is necessary to be interested in the activities about us. Those who think of nothing or no one except themselves are almost dead to the world, even though they go through the same physical activities as other people. The tendency is to get into a rut with advancing years and remain there. It is easy to keep both a pliable mind and a pliable body in spite of age, and this can be done by intelligent use. A short time daily should be spent in becoming informed of what is happening throughout the world and thinking it over. A mental hobby is most excellent. A garden or a few birds can furnish an almost inexhaustible source of interest. Those who doubt this should read of the comedy and tragedy among such humble beings as the spider, the fly and the beetle. J. H. Fabre has written charmingly about these, investing them with an interest rarely to be found in good fiction. This naturalist is a good example of what can be accomplished when one has years to do it in and is content to labor along from day to day without giving too much thought for the morrow. At fifty Mr. Fabre was practically unknown. Now, at about ninety, he is one of the most admired and best loved of men. His recognition came late and he has done much of his best work during his later years. If Mr. Fabre had died at the average age of forty, the world would have been deprived of his beautiful insight.

Another cause of old age is getting mentally old. An individual begins to grow old by dwelling on the subject. The girl of thirteen must cease romping and racing about because it is not lady-like. At twenty-five it is very, very undignified to run a little. At forty a woman must be rather sedate, for being natural would mean frivolity. People are continually growing too old to do this and that, not because they have lost the desire and the ability, but because it is unbecoming at their age. This is folly. Keep a young heart all through life. A heartfelt laugh is one of nature's best tonics. There is no more harm in dancing at fifty than at fifteen and not so much danger.

The relaxation of muscles and sagging of the face are as much the result of mental attitude as of loss of tonicity. Thinking young and associating with children are helpful and healthful. People who are very stiff and dignified are mentally sterile. The charming people are the ones who are willing and able to understand and sympathize with the aims and aspirations of others, and in order to do so it is necessary to thaw out.

The art of life is delightful if properly developed.

Worry is such a detriment that its victims can neither live nor work as they should. It is necessary to overcome this bad habit. Most of the worry is due to narrow selfishness. Much of it is caused by the fact that others will not do as we do. To try to make others accept our standards and then worry and fret because they will not is folly. When force is employed to convert anyone the conversion is but superficial and lasts only so long as the converted individual's hypocrisy holds out. To get the best out of life we have to be broad, forbearing, patient and forgiving.

A normal old age is beautiful. It is the privilege, nay more, the duty of every intelligent being to attain it. When we adjust ourselves we shall live longer.

It is with old age as it is with health. We can have it if we wish it. Accidents alone can deprive us of either. Let us hope that the day will come when men and women will not be satisfied to die as life is but beginning, but that they will live as they should and could live, thus proving a blessing to the race.

CHAPTER XXIX.

EVOLVING INTO HEALTH.

By the time most people are twenty years old they have some kind of disease. It may be only a slight catarrh, a touch of indigestion, trouble with the eyes, defective hearing, or some other ill. Very seldom do we meet a person of this age who is perfectly well.

Most people are taught to believe that health is something mysterious which may come to them or may pass them by, but that they have little or nothing to do with it. If they are well, they are fortunate, but if they are ill they are not to blame.

Most of them go to conventional physicians when they are ill, expecting to be cured. They take medicine or injections of serums or they are operated upon. When they are through with the doctors they are no wiser than they were before.

A few have friends who tell them that they must change their mode of living if they would have health. They are interested enough to go to a healer who believes in nature. He tells them that they are well or ill according to their desserts, that they can be well at all times, if they wish, for if they live as they should health is a natural consequence.

This sounds like nonsense at first. It is different from anything else they have heard. The sufferer often makes up his mind that the healer is a fool or a faker. He remembers that when he went to the conventional physicians they sounded and thumped him and examined all his excretions. They were very thorough and scientific. The natural healer does not generally go into so many details. He asks enough and examines enough to find the trouble and then he stops. This the patient charges against him, for he takes for granted that the healer is brief from lack of knowledge.

So he goes back to his old physician. As his trouble is due to deranged nutrition, he does not get well. He thinks over what the natural healer said, and the more he thinks about it the more reasonable it sounds, and he returns again. This time he gets instructions, and he follows them enough to get benefit, but not faithfully enough to get well. He is convinced that the conventional physicians are wrong, but still believes that the natural healer can hardly be right.

After a while he makes up his mind to get down to business and he goes to the healer for instructions and follows them. The results are surprising. The trouble he has had for years may disappear within a month or two, or it may become less and less apparent, but take considerable time before it leaves entirely.

The healer gives instructions. The most important ones are those concerning the diet. A plan is given that brings good results. The healer fails to explain that this is but one correct method of feeding, that there are other good ones. The patient is enthused over the benefits derived, he makes up his mind that he is living the only correct life, and he too often becomes a food crank, trying to force his ideas upon all about him. Here the healer is at fault, for he should explain that some method is necessary, but that there is no one and only method of feeding.

If the patient is fairly intelligent, in time he realizes that it is not so much what he eats as his manner of eating and moderation that are helpful, and that any plan in which moderation and simplicity are followed is better than the ordinary way of eating.

As the patient evolves into health and gets a broader view of the art of living, he gets a better perspective of life. He learns that under like conditions like causes always produce like effects, that the law of compensation is always operative, and we therefore get what we deserve. He loses his fear of many things that caused him grave concern previously. He sees in sickness and death the working of natural law, not of chance.

Some patients realize that healers who work in accordance with nature are right, at the very start, but most people are not so logically constructed. It often takes from one to three years before people make up their mind to order their lives so that they can have health at their command.

In the old way, the doctor was supposed to cure, which was impossible. In the new way, the healer educates people and then if they live their knowledge they get health.

The healer must instruct in the care of all parts of the body, weeding out bad habits and trying to instill good ones in their place.

Eating according to correct principles is the most helpful and powerful aid in regaining health. The patient finds that as the years pass his tastes change, becoming more simple and more moderate. He is well nourished on one-half to one-third of what he used to consume and consider necessary.

The following is the last half of a month's record of food intake for a man in the thirties. Some years ago he changed his manner of living in order to regain health, in which he succeeded. Now he takes only one or two meals a day, according to his desires, not that he has any objection to three meals a day, but he finds it best to eat more seldom. He is in good physical condition, as heavy as he ought to be, and he has not had any real physical trouble for a number of years. His work is mental, but he walks considerably and swims from three to six times a week, besides taking a few set exercises.

It was taken in spring, the weather averaging cool. This is a little lighter than usual, because the record was taken during a period of exceptionally hard mental work. In cold weather heavier foods are taken.

Lunch: Nothing.

Dinner: Three slices of rye toast, very thin, celery, three slices broiled onion, dish of peas, glass of beer.

Dinner at noon: Roast lamb, dish of spinach, one and one-half dishes summer squash, lettuce and tomato salad.

Supper: Nothing.

Lunch: Dish of baked lentils, vegetable soup, lettuce.

Dinner: Two small oranges, cottage cheese.

Lunch: Piece of gingerbread, cup of cocoa, two lumps of sugar.

Dinner: Two small oranges, cottage cheese.

Lunch: Dish of stewed prunes, tablespoonful cottage cheese.

Dinner: Two eggs, two slices buttered toast.

Lunch: Small grapefruit.

Dinner: Vegetable soup, dish of stewed turnips, dish of peas.

Lunch: Nothing.

Dinner: Half a grapefruit, three stewed figs, glass of milk.

Lunch: Dish of strawberries, large dish of rhubarb with grapefruit juice in it and cream on the side; half serving cream cheese.

Dinner: Two small baked apples.

Lunch: Small grapefruit.

Dinner: Two eggs, dish of turnips, dish of spinach, sliced tomatoes.

Lunch: One raw apple.

Dinner: Two shredded wheat biscuits, glass of milk.

Lunch: Dish of rhubarb.

Dinner: Vegetable soup, one egg, a boiled potato.

Lunch: Dish of rhubarb.

Dinner: Sweet potato, dish of parsnips, stewed peas.

Lunch: Dish of ice cream, piece of white cake. Dinner: Cheese cake, dish of fruit salad.

Lunch: One hard boiled egg, about one and one-half slices white bread, two big radishes, one young onion, butter.

Dinner: Nothing.

The servings are the ordinary restaurant servings. No dressings were used except the ones mentioned. This man used to be very fond of sweets and employed salt freely. Now he finds his foods more agreeable when taken plain, for they have a better flavor. He rarely uses salt or pepper. He has simplified his food intake because he finds he feels better and stronger and is able to think to better advantage than he did when he partook of a greater variety and amount of food at each meal.

Food scientists say that from two thousand, seven hundred to three thousand, three hundred calories are needed daily, but you will note that this man generally keeps below one-half of this, if you are able to figure food values.

People who are trying to get well are often called fools and cranks when they treat themselves properly, but this does not matter, for such fools generally live to see their wise critics prematurely consigned to the earth.

When taking health advice, try to keep your balance. Get thoroughly well before you try to guide others.

CHAPTER XXX.

RETROSPECT.

Several hundred pages have been devoted to those matters which must receive attention in order to have good physical and mental health, so as to be able to get the most out of life and give the most, that is, in order to live fully. The basis of health is internal cleanliness, and to attain this it is necessary to exercise self-control and moderation, as well as to cultivate good will and kindliness towards others. Kindness and love lubricate life and make the running smooth. Envy, spite, hatred and the other negative emotions act like sand in the bearings, producing friction in the vital machinery, which they destroy in the end.

Success in life means balance, poise, adjustment. We must adjust ourselves so as to be in harmony with others, and we must be in harmony with nature. Our minds will at times be in opposition to the laws of nature. Then we must exercise enough self-control to bring them into harmony again, for natural laws are no respecters of persons. It is said that we break these laws, but that is not true. If we disregard them often enough they break us. We must realize our unity with nature, our at-one-ment. We must realize that we are a part of nature, not above it, and hence that we are governed by the same fixed laws that govern the rest of nature. These laws are for our good. Attempts to escape from their workings indicate a lack of understanding.

Discord produces disease and death. Harmony leads to health and long life.

The adjustment must be both physical and mental.

The physical part means to live or adjust ourselves so that all the functions of the body are carried on normally. The body is self-regulating and if we do nothing harmful health will be our portion. However, life under our present civilization is so complex that the demands upon our nervous systems are excessive. It is easy to live so that we can have health, but to do so is not conventional, and hence not very popular.

In order to have good physical health under present conditions, it is necessary to make some effort. The effort is not great enough to be onerous and does not require much time. It is important to get health knowledge, which the majority lacks today. This knowledge is most excellent, but it does not benefit the individual unless it is applied. We all wish to have health, but this is not enough. We must will to have it. When we say that we cannot, it should generally be interpreted to mean that we will not.

Some important subjects regarding which special knowledge should be secured are: Food, drink, exercise, care of the skin, sleep, work and play, breathing, clothing, and mental attitude.

These subjects, as well as others, have been quite extensively discussed. It is impossible to give full information in tabloid form. It is also impossible to read a book of this character once and get all the information it contains. Those who are in earnest will study the subject, instead of merely reading it.

Allow me to remind you that nearly all of our diseases are due to faulty dietary habits. So it was in the time of Hippocrates, according to that sage, and so it is today. It is a common statement that about 90 per cent. of our physical ills come from improper diet, and this is the truth. It follows from this that it is most important to know about correct feeding habits, and put them in practice. Improper diet results in faulty nutrition, after which physical and mental ills make their appearance.

There are many systems of feeding, and nearly all of them will bring good results if the most important prescription is followed, namely, moderation. Simplicity leads to moderation.

Those who are reasonable about their food intake often serve as targets for the shafts of ridicule launched at them by those who are ignorant of the subject or too self-indulgent to exercise a little self-control. Ridicule is one of the most deadly of weapons, but it never harms those who have the hardihood of getting down to basic facts and classifying things and ideas according to their true value. Why should we be guided by the wit and sarcasm of indolent voluptuaries who daily desecrate their bodies through ruinous indulgences?

There is no need of becoming harsh and austere, nor is it necessary to fall into deadly habits of self-indulgence. Sometimes we can go with the current with benefit, but at times it is also necessary to paddle up-stream. Life demands a certain amount of hardihood from those who would live in health, and this comes not from self-indulgence, but from self-denial. It is necessary to do almost daily something that we are not inclined to do.

It is well to remember that if the eating is correct, it is difficult to become physically deranged, and consequently to become mentally deranged. Allow me to repeat four short sentences which are helpful and most important guides, sentences which ought to form a part of every child's education:

If ill, eat nothing, but live on water.

Eat only when there is a desire for food.

Masticate all foods thoroughly.

Always be moderate in your food intake.

These are the four golden rules regarding eating, and if they were adhered to, they would save us from an incalculable amount of sin and suffering. They would increase the duration of life and the joy of living. They would add to our physical and mental prosperity. Hence they are worthy of the emphasis given them.

In brief: Physical health is based on internal cleanliness, which can be attained only through moderation, that is, by not habitually overburdening the system, especially with food. Our bodies thrive when used, but not when abused. It is necessary for our physical well-being to get air, sunshine, water, food, sleep, rest, exercise, work and play in proper proportion, and in addition cultivate a kindly, balanced spirit. Drugs, such as alcohol, coffee, morphine, bromine, and hundreds of others which could be named, are not only unnecessary, but harmful.

The mental side is as important as the physical side. With a healthy body it is easy to have a happy outlook. Indigestion and biliousness can make a dreary waste out of the most beautiful landscape. The body and mind react and interact, one upon the other. When one is poised it is easy to get the other into balance. It requires a poised body to produce the best fruitage--a fine spirit.

It is necessary to be honest with one's self. Face life courageously and honestly. If you do, you will soon realize that the physical and mental ills from which you suffer are mostly of your own making. Then you can choose whether to let them continue or to end them, but if you choose to remain ill, bear your cross uncomplainingly, for you have no right to afflict others with your self-imposed sufferings.

On the other hand, try to see life from the view point of others, and you will often find that what you think is the highest good and most desirable in life does not seem worthy of great effort to them. Variety adds spice to life. To impose one's own views and ways on others has always seemed desirable to the majority of people, but it is the height of folly and stupidity. So long as the race exists there will be many men of many minds, and it is best so. We can not force any benefit, such as health or goodness, upon others. Instead of attracting, the process of forcing repels.

What we can do mentally to benefit ourselves and others is to get adjusted, to cultivate kindness and charity, to be broad-minded and forgiving, to be slow to take and give offense, to accept the little buffetings that fate has in store for us all with good grace, and through it all to possess our souls in patience.

Physically, be moderate.

Mentally, cultivate equanimity.

###